D0282660

RT 86.7 .P83 1983

Puetz, Belinda E.

Networking for nurses

Fairleigh Dickinson University Library
Teaneck, New Jersey

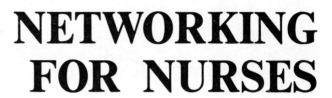

NETWORKING FOR NURSES

Belinda E. Puetz, R.N., Ph.D.

Indiana State Nurses Association

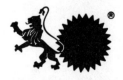

AN ASPEN PUBLICATION®
Aspen Systems Corporation
Rockville, Maryland
London
1983

RT
86.7
.P83
1983

Library of Congress Cataloging in Publication Data

Puetz, Belinda E.
Networking for nurses.

Includes bibliographical references and index.
1. Nurses—Employment. 2. Women's networks.
3. Nursing—Vocational guidance. I. Title.
[DNLM: 1. Career mobility—Nursing texts. 2. Inter-
professional relations—Nursing texts. WY 16 P977n]
RT86.7.P83   1983   610.73'06'9   82-20669
ISBN: 0-89443-670-8

Fairleigh Dickinson
University Library

TEANECK, NEW JERSEY

Publisher: John Marozsan
Editorial Director: Darlene Como
Managing Editor: Margot Raphael
Editorial Services: Eileen Higgins
Printing and Manufacturing: Debbie Collins

Copyright © 1983 by Aspen Systems Corporation

All rights reserved. This book, or parts thereof, may not be
reproduced in any form or by any means, electronic or
mechanical, including photocopy, recording, or any
information storage and retrieval system now known or
to be invented, without written permission from the
publisher, except in the case of brief quotations embodied
in critical articles or reviews. For information, address
Aspen Systems Corporation, 1600 Research Boulevard,
Rockville, Maryland 20850.

Library of Congress Catalog Card Number: 82-20669
ISBN: 0-89443-670-8

Printed in the United States of America

1 2 3 4 5

06/16/83   22.50

To all those who were or who are now part of my professional network: *Ruth L. Johnston, Grace L. Penrod, John McKinley, Jean E. Schweer,* the late *H. Walton Connelly, Faye L. Peters,* my brother, *William J. Puetz,* and, most of all, my husband, *Werner F. Kuhn.* These, and many others, are among those caring people who have helped me along the way.

Table of Contents

Foreword

As the author of this book readily tells you, there is nothing new about the concept of networking as a useful technique in moving up the career ladder. And even though men have the reputation of using the system effectively for their own advancement, women have been doing a lot of quiet, unidentified networking as well. Nurses, too, have had (and used) their professional networks.

My own nursing career (as opposed to job) started when a night supervisor with whom I developed a friendship recommended me for a teaching position and strongly urged me to take this new step. And, as a young teacher, I was firmly directed by an older colleague to attend nursing meetings, regardless of my personal priorities, because making professional "contacts" was essential. She was right. In more than two decades of attending meetings, I found I wasn't the only one who had a dual purpose.

Yet, only a short while ago, after a version of that little story was published in a national journal, I was taken to task by a well-known nurse. According to that individual, it just wasn't legitimate to use professional meetings for anything other than their educational or organizational purpose. Because there still are many individuals who feel like this, *Networking for Nurses* is not only timely but can also make a real contribution to nursing.

Whether or not some nurses (or perhaps to a minor extent, all nurses) use networking to achieve certain goals, the potential lies untapped. As long as nurse networking is relatively unacknowledged, unidentified, underutilized, and worst, unrespected, we are dissipating our energies in trying to affect health care policy. We can have only limited impact if we don't have enough knowledgeable nurses in key positions.

Thus, the nurse influentials, as Vance[1] calls them, must first arrive, and then be ready and willing to play a leadership role (with a well-developed network). There's more to networking than networking, and this book points the way.

To begin with, Puetz provides the fundamental concepts of networking. The next two chapters which address how to use networking and how to start a network can prove particularly helpful to both students and graduates on the way up. Since much that is written about networking seems to focus on the one-to-one relationships or the expansion of existing networks, the discussion of how to create a network to meet a specific need is not only refreshing, but eminently practical.

I must admit that my favorite chapter is on mentoring, since I have a special commitment to being a mentor and have had the advantage and privilege of being "mentored" by a nursing leader early in my career. The hows and whats are discussed comprehensively and lucidly, but anyone who has been either protégé or mentor will particularly appreciate the call for nurses to give more attention to the importance of mentorship. Being a mentor is a serious and time consuming responsibility, but more of our nurse influentials must assume this role. And for those potential protégés who have not been chosen, the advice on how to take the initiative is extremely useful and, of course, necessary.

Equally useful are the chapters by Shinn identifying strategies for using networks both to gain political influence and to become effective when involved in labor relations. There is a great deal of information in these chapters that goes beyond simple networking (if networking is ever simple), again emphasizing the need to be knowledgeable about what one is involved with before trying to use a network.

Probably many nurses have not thought of the importance of developing themselves in every sense, as a part of the networking technique; yet marketing yourself is a must. The concluding chapter addresses other strategies for professional growth and looks at networking from a broader perspective, pointing the way to further self-development and growth.

There is no question that *Networking for Nurses* will be valuable for the young nurse or the one who has just become career and profession oriented. It is readable, pragmatic, and multifaceted. Yet it also has useful

[1]Connie Vance, "A Group Profile of Contemporary Influentials in American Nursing." Ed.D. Dissertation, Teachers College, Columbia University, 1977.

information for an experienced networker. Most of all, it should enable nurses to initiate or enhance their networking skill.

Lucie S. Kelly, R.N., Ph.D., F.A.A.N.
Professor of Public Health in
Health Administration
and Nursing
Columbia University

Preface

Become Cinderella instead of Sleeping Beauty. The difference between Sleeping Beauty and Cinderella is that Sleeping Beauty slept for a hundred years. Cinderella got up in the morning and got out of bed. She got dressed. She used her stepsisters . . . to give her information about a very key event. Then, she plugged in to her mentor, the fairy godmother, who had resources (little animals and a pumpkin) that were utilized on her behalf. When she got to the ball, she was imaged appropriately and knew how to dance. And then, she knew when to leave.

—Alina Novak
Keynote address, the 1981 Annual Conference
on Continuing Education in Nursing,
American Nurses' Association Council on
Continuing Education, Washington, D.C.

This volume is the result of the networking process. At the 1981 Annual Conference of the American Nurses' Association Council on Continuing Education, I had the distinct pleasure of listening to a keynote address by Alina Novak. Alina described the concepts of networking and, in a fun-filled hour, encouraged us to identify our existing networks.

Afterwards, in the coffee shop, several of us talked about networking and what it meant, or could mean, to nurses. We talked about how we had gotten to where we were in our careers—who had helped us, and, in turn, whom we were helping. And then, I thought, how much easier my path to success would have been with a mentor, and with established networks, rather than the "hit and miss" methods I used, for lack of any better ones. Someone suggested that nurses needed to know more about networking, and the idea for *Networking for Nurses* was born.

Through networking with my nurse colleagues, I determined that there was a real need for the book. There also was a sense of excitement about the possibility of such a book.

During a trip to the Soviet Union in November of 1981, I tried the idea of a networking book out on Fitzhugh Mullan, M.D., one of the members of the health care delegation with whom I was traveling. He was enthusiastic and provided many of the ideas that are incorporated in the book. Another member of our delegation, Lucie S. Kelly, Ph.D., stressed the real need for mentors in nursing, and stimulated many thoughts on the process of helping as well as being helped.

Thus, my original ideas for *Networking for Nurses* took form. Other colleagues provided the moral support and encouragement necessary during the writing of the book. Particularly helpful was Margaret de Boer, who guided me through the vagaries of working with a computer word-processing program. Also, Linda J. Shinn, who contributed two chapters, deserves thanks for her assistance and support.

The concept of networking is relatively new to nursing. Since most nurses are women, the focus of this book is on female nurses networking with one another and with other members of the health care team. Male nurses were not deliberately omitted. Networking can be, and is, as useful to men as it is to women. Men, however, have less need for a book to tell them how to network. Men have been socialized from their early days to network successfully with others. Women in general are just now learning about networking with other women, and nurses specifically are therefore learning how to network. *Networking for Nurses* is intended to make the process of learning to network, or improving existing networking skills, a bit easier for nurses.

Some nurses look upon networking as the latest of many "fads" to affect the profession. Without the real support and assistance from others, however, many of those who disdain networking would not be where they are today in their professional lives.

The examples used in the book are taken from real situations, or composites of those situations. The names of the nurses in those situations have been changed, but the individuals portrayed represent nurses everywhere.

Belinda E. Puetz
December 1982

Chapter 1

What Networking Is

Networking is nothing new; it always existed. Networking existed primarily in the male-oriented business world. Networking occurred in the dining rooms of athletic and other private clubs, in sports facilities such as racquetball or tennis clubs, on the golf links, in pools, saunas, and in locker rooms. Networking activities weren't just confined to such leisure pastimes. Networking also occurred in the corridors, offices, cafeterias, and parking lots of business establishments across the nation. Men used their networks to get ahead.

In *Webster's New World Dictionary*, a network is defined as "(1) Any arrangement of fabric or parallel wires, threads etc., crossed at regular intervals by others fastened to them so as to leave open spaces. (2) A system of interconnected or cooperating individuals."

The system men used was called the "old boys' network." The old boys' network was comprised of acquaintances, colleagues, and friends from all over—school, church, family, sports, and business. When a man needed something he contacted one of the other old boys—over lunch, dinner, or drinks. The contact could also be made over a tennis net or over the telephone.

Using such contacts seems to be an automatic response on the part of businessmen. Men grow up knowing how to network, partially because of the emphasis on team sports during a boy's formative years. Boys learn how to collaborate, to help one another for the good of the team. They learn not to hold grudges. They learn quickly and well that they need one another in order to win the game, to get ahead.

These boys then grow into men who have learned that they need their colleagues in order to achieve what they want in the world of business. Whether or not they like their teammates, they are a team, working together for the common good. And, if self-interest can be served as well as the interest of the group, all the better for the individual.

1

The end result of this socialization process that leads to such effective old boys' networks is that men obtain what they want or need in business. Using such contacts to get ahead, to climb up the corporate ladder of success, has been reserved for men—until recently.

Women began entering the world of business in greater numbers and at higher levels as a result of the Women's Movement. These women noticed that their path to the top often was not as smooth as that of their male counterparts.

Enterprising feminists attempted to assess the reasons for this discrepancy. One of the main reasons, they discovered, was that there was no "old girls' network" similar to the old boys' networks for men, which women could use in order to achieve their professional goals.

Part of the reason for the absence of an old girls' network is that women are not socialized into team sports as youngsters. Women learning to compete learn only as individuals; they learn how to distrust others, particularly other women, with whom they are in competition. Men, on the other hand, learn that compromise, collaboration, and cooperation are important components of competition.

Women in the business world are in competition with one another and with men for advancement. These women are finding that they do not have the access they need to personal recommendations for key positions in business or for assuming responsibility for a special project within their employing agency.

In the not too distant past, as women entered formerly male-dominated fields of employment, they found they didn't have access to vital information needed to conduct business: they didn't know who the crucial approval would need to come from; they didn't know who had the final say in documenting a suggested change; they didn't know who to approach for information that was classified as "secret."

Perhaps most important, they didn't know the necessary strategies for doing what they needed to do on their jobs: they didn't know how to sell the president on the proposed changes; they didn't know that it is the secretary in the Personnel Office who will release the necessary financial records for review; and they didn't know that it's far more efficient to approach the Research and Development Department first than to wait until they come to you having heard rumors that a project is underway. Knowing the right people would have provided this information for women as the old boys' network had provided similar kinds of information for men.

Women who previously had been content to get ahead "on their own," although it was an arduous process, began to appreciate the advantages of making and using contacts. They "called in favors" from other women they had met over bridge, at Parent-Teacher Association (PTA) meetings, or in church. In turn, other women called on them.

Soon, these women realized that over time they had established a large number of individual contacts to whom they could turn for information, advice, support, or access to others. Understanding the significance of these contacts as one way to get ahead was enlightening to many women in business and served as the basis for the birth of networking by and for women.

Information about women's networks and the concept and process of networking began appearing in the feminist literature in the late 70s. Simply put, women's networks came about because they were needed and needed urgently by women.

TYPES OF NETWORKS

There are many kinds of women's networks. In her recent book titled *Women's Networks,* Carol Kleinman lists 1,400 national and local networks.[1] There are networks for every interest area known to women. Networks have been formed of women who like to cook (the Gourmet Exchange) and those who hate cooking (Pillsbury Bake-Off Girls). There are networks for women who like running, race walking, or other sports. Women are forming networks with each other based on age, or marital status, such as being widowed or divorced.

There are networks for single parents and for those experiencing various emotional crises, such as runaway teens, or children with drug or alcohol problems. Women who meet together to share experiences and support one another through recovery from a mastectomy are networking. There are networks for abused women.

In addition to networks for women in business or in the professions, there are networks for political action. There are networks for women in government, at the local, state, and national levels. There are networks for women in the arts, for women who live in rural areas, for women in the labor movement, for women in the social sciences, and for women in various religious groups.

These are only a few of the types of existing networks. More networks are being formed every day as women realize how valuable they are and how successful networking efforts are.

WHY NETWORK?

Networking, as defined by Mary Scott Welch, author of the book *Networking,* is "the process of developing and using your contacts for information, advice and moral support as you pursue your career."[2] Networks are being established by women today for the express purpose of helping themselves and one another.

Networking provides for women in business a sense of having mastered the system. When women use their networks to move through the system in a smooth, orderly fashion, they have the feeling of accomplishment. Where before their progress was accompanied by a feeling of "fighting the system," now they move ahead by using the system to their advantage.

Women who network effectively also have a greater sense of self-worth. Networking enhances one's self-esteem. When others include us in their networks and seek our advice and counsel we tend to feel better about ourselves and our worth.

Networking, however, is not a one-way street. Women who network not only get from other women, they give. When women communicate together for the achievement of their professional goals they provide ever larger networks for themselves and for other women. They refer each other to still other contacts who subsequently become part of an expanding network. They seek help from others in advancing their own careers, but also offer help to those whose careers they can help.

NETWORKING APPLIED TO NURSING

Women don't network exclusively with women; many of the best contacts in a woman's network are men. But, because this book is devoted to the concept of networking applied to nursing, the techniques described will be those necessary and appropriate for networking in a primarily female profession.

Networking to get ahead in nursing is an idea that is relatively new and not yet very well accepted. The idea that nurses might want to "get ahead," that they are ambitious, is still somewhat unsettling to those who visualize nurses as nurturing, caring, passive, and dependent individuals.

The idea that networkers "use" people also is difficult for some women to deal with. "But, that's manipulating people," some say. Realistically speaking, we all learn to manipulate others early in life. From the time we first say "no" to something mother tells us to do (and get away with it), we learn to get what we want from others.

In a normal, healthy person, manipulation is used for the purpose of getting needs met. Those persons who manipulate only to get others to do what they want are exploiting others for their own personal gain. Such a person manipulates to control others' behavior rather than to meet personal needs. That is not a normal, healthy use of manipulation.[3]

In networking, contacts are used to help get us what we want or need. Other individuals in our networks use us in turn to get what they want or need. This use of individuals by each other, although manipulation by definition, is appropriate and perfectly normal.

Common sense tells us that effectively using the informal contacts within an institution or organization is important. Even if an individual has all it takes to get ahead, it doesn't hurt to have a recommendation to ease the passage up. In most instances, although there are exceptions, if an individual doesn't have the necessary competence, no amount of referrals will assist in his or her career advancement.

We've all heard the cliché "It's not what you know, but who you know that counts." In networking, those informal contacts are used. Contacts will help an individual move up the ladder of success, assuming that the individual's basic performance will permit such advancement.

Networking has payoffs on both sides. As you use people to get what you want, you will find that they, in turn, will use you. The arrangement is reciprocal. You may not ever be in a position to return a favor to someone who did you a favor. But you certainly will be in a position to pass the favor along to someone else. The favor you do for someone else may not be as significant as the favor you received. The need for you to return the favor may not occur immediately after you receive your favor. Nonetheless, despite occasional discrepancies, there is an exchange of benefits in the networking process.

Even those nurses who are relatively comfortable with their present state can benefit through the application of networking skills in their professional life. The nurse reading this book may wish only to attain a promotion, or learn to be more assertive with a troublesome co-worker or physician. On the other hand, the reader may wish to use networking to advance his or her career or to seek and obtain a new job, or to participate in the enactment of legislation to which he or she is professionally committed, or to serve as a catalyst in organizing the nurses with whom he or she works for the purpose of negotiating their wages, hours, and working conditions.

Networking applies to all nurses in all areas of nursing practice. It is the individual nurse who will decide to what extent he or she wishes to use the techniques of networking. Using the techniques of networking in no way implies that the nurse agrees with or supports the feminist movement. Networking is not a commitment to a larger cause, the adoption of a militant posture toward women's issues, or the unhealthy manipulation of others to get one's own way. Networking allows nurses to take advantage of those contacts they already have and to effectively expand those contacts in order to assist in meeting their professional goals. Networking can be an asset to the nurse that in no way must result in the compromise of his or her professional ideals and principles.

HOW NURSES NETWORK

Nurses network now; they use their professional and personal contacts to get what they want. For example, in a typical interchange, a nurse says to a colleague, "I've had a bad time with Dr. Jones again today. He just doesn't seem to understand that I'm also responsible for the health care his patients receive. I feel I have to tell him when I think a new drug I've read about could be more effective with one of his patients. He just tells me I'm interfering, that he's in charge of his patients' treatment plan. What do you think?"

This is an example of a nurse who is seeking information, advice, and/or moral support from a colleague. She is networking. When her colleague responds, "I don't really know what to tell you; I haven't had much experience with Dr. Jones. Mary Marvin on nights has worked with him longer than either one of us; let's ask her advice," the network has been expanded even further.

When Mary further helps the nurse in our example by involving her in the local nurses' group that meets to discuss mutual concerns about patient care, the network has been expanded even further. Thus, the nurse in this illustration uses her network for information, advice, and moral support, assisting her in meeting her professional goal of quality patient care.

In another typical example, a nurse asks for advice from a friend: "Say, can you take a look at this memo on the proposed new absenteeism policy? Does it really look like I'm interested in people's comments? I sure don't want to make anybody think this is an accomplished fact already; I really want some input. This is my first supervisory position and I don't want people thinking I'm just issuing orders with this memo!"

Again, as in our previous example, this nurse is using her existing network to achieve a goal. In this instance, the nurse's acceptance as a supervisor by those whom she supervises and her ultimate promotion to higher levels of nursing management could well benefit from her use of networking techniques.

Networking is an effective strategy for women to use in attempting to make their way in the male-dominated work world. While nursing is a primarily female profession (98 percent of practicing nurses are women), many of those individuals with whom the female nurse must work, particularly persons in positions of authority, such as hospital administrators and physicians, are men.

Most nurses, like women in general, work because they must. Women traditionally have the lowest-paying positions, despite the fact that there are more of them in the work world than there are men. The most recent statistics indicate that women working full time earn 59 cents for every dollar earned by men. Unfortunately, despite the feminist movement and affirmative action programs, the gap between men's and women's wages is increasing rather than decreasing.[4]

Traditionally, women also have the lowest-level jobs. Nursing has been considered by many to be an occupation rather than a profession; only the militant and vocal efforts of some nursing leaders have elevated the status of nursing in recent years. Despite the fact that nurses comprise the largest segment of the population of health care workers, they are not highly regarded.

Increasingly, nurses are realizing that it will take a conscious and concerted effort to change the image of nursing and the conditions under which nurses work. Nurses are recognizing that the system must change in order for the profession of nursing to come into its own. The system is resistant to change, particularly change based on change efforts typically employed by women (and nurses). Networking provides a means for nurses, as well as others, to work within the existing constraints of the system to attain their goals.

HOW NETWORKING WORKS

Networking is largely an information-exchanging process between individuals. Networkers check with one another for advice about problems, for referrals to sources of assistance, for recommendations, and/or for feedback about personal and professional situations. Finally, networkers who are mentors to others assist them to get ahead.

Networking works for nurses as it works for women in general. The concept, process, and skills of networking apply in the nursing profession as they do in all areas of women's employment.

An illustration of networking between two women employed in an industry might be as follows:

> I got the promotion offer; isn't that great? They gave me until Monday to decide. One thing bothers me, though. My raise will bring me to $17,500 a year. Rumor has it that when there was a man in this position he was making $22,500. Know anything about that? Can you check it out on your end for me? Thanks; I appreciate it.

A typical networking exchange in nursing might be:

> I understand you're trying out the new decubitus care routine that you learned at the continuing education offering last month. How is it working for you?
> Or:
> We're getting together this evening to discuss a plan for proposing a new work schedule in the critical care units. We thought we'd like to try the 10-hour shift, 4-day work week. Would you like to join us? Do you know anyone else who might be interested?
> Or, still another:
> I understand there's going to be a position open soon for a coordinator of the baccalaureate program. I wondered if anyone teaching in the junior year might be interested?
> And, one final example:
> I just got a request for a workshop on basic supervisory skills at County Hospital. I understand Dan Matthews, the chief nurse at the Visiting Nurses' Association, taught for you last year on the same topic. How was he? Would you recommend him to teach a similar program for me?

These examples of networking should be familiar; they occur in everyday conversation for most of us. Each of these exchanges took place for a definite purpose. The person seeking the information had a reason for initiating the interchange. Whether the purpose is for information, feedback, or to give or get a referral, nurses can use networking to accomplish their goals.

Nurses also will find networking skills useful in helping others accomplish their goals, as in the following example:

> Suzanne, this is Monica. Great game last night! Your backhand is getting terrific! Say, I called to find out if you are still looking for someone to head the research project on hypertension you just had funded? I've got someone to recommend to you: Marcie Sills just finished her doctorate and is looking for a position for a year or two until her husband has completed his dissertation when they'll be moving back out west. She has the research skills; that was her minor during her graduate work. And I can attest to her administrative ability when she worked for me several years ago as head of the department. Want to know how to get in touch with her?

Such examples illustrate the similarity between networking in other areas of women's employment and networking in nursing. It can be seen that the principles of networking apply equally to women whether employed in business, industry, or nursing.

SUCCESS IN NETWORKING

Most networking success stories, however, have been reported by women other than nurses. In an article published in the magazine of the Life Office Management Association, *Resource,* Alina Novak, senior financial analyst for the Equitable Life Assurance Society of the United States, described her networking experiences.[5] She began as an administrative assistant at Equitable, one employee among thousands. Although Equitable had an affirmative action program that provided special activities for the women employees, Alina felt they weren't meeting the specific needs of women in the company to get ahead. Most of the activities were planned and implemented for the women employees rather than by them.

Alina decided to change that and began meeting with her friends in the company to see if they felt as she did. She expanded her circle of contacts and found that many of the women with whom she spoke shared thoughts and feelings similar to hers. When Alina was ready to "go public" with her ideas, she arranged a meeting and many of the women with whom she'd had private discussions came. The issues raised at the meeting led the group to realize that it was important to decide where to go next. Thus, the network at Equitable was begun.

Alina Novak now is a recognized expert on networking. She appears regularly on television and on the lecture circuit because of her past and current networking activities. She effectively and enthusiastically personifies networking success.

Another instance of networking success was reported in *Time* magazine.[6] That article described several women who noted that more than one-third of the candidates for master's degrees in Business Administration are women. Yet, none of the women in executive positions in corporations are members of the all-male organization The Business Roundtable. Accordingly, they organized their own group, called the Committee of 200.

The Committee of 200 is described as a "national women's business group with a national focus." There are specific membership criteria for the group: the woman has to be in charge of the business, either entirely or to a large extent and the company must have annual sales of $5 million or more. A woman executive who manages a budget of $5 million also is eligible for membership.

Of the 1,400 women who met those standards, only 40 percent elected to join the Committee of 200. Interestingly, many women were concerned about the relationship of the group to "women's rights" issues or admitted being too "work-oriented" to be able to focus on much outside of their work activities.

Those women who elected to join the Committee of 200 appeared pleased after the initial meeting of the group, in early April 1982. Many of the comments made by those in attendance reflected their surprise that they had female colleagues with similar problems. Others indicated they experienced support from the group, receiving both reinforcement for their individual success in attaining the positions they held and for their abilities to deal with the stresses associated with those positions.

The Committee of 200 is primarily a forum for the exchange of opinions and views of these very successful businesswomen. Education of the members appears to be an integral component of the group's focus. The group plans regional sessions throughout the United States as well as future national meetings.

Thus, another network of women is formed. The women attending the initial meeting of the Committee of 200 described, in their comments after the meeting, many of the benefits and advantages of successful networking groups.

WHEN NETWORKING DOESN'T WORK

Not all networking stories are stories of success. Occasionally, networking doesn't work. Most often the reason for failure is that networking wasn't used when it should have been, as in an instance when the woman wasn't aware of what was going on in the employment setting which ultimately affected her.

For example, Sylvia Morgan is a newly employed psychiatric nurse in the out-patient clinic of a comprehensive mental health center. The center's director is a psychologist, and the chief of clinical services for both the in- and out-patient services is a psychiatrist. Sylvia feels that she is clinically prepared to conduct therapy with clients on an individual or group basis. The psychiatrist feels that Sylvia's work should be closely supervised by a physician. There are other individuals involved in therapy with the center's clients, but they are social workers. Sylvia is the first nurse employed in the role of therapist.

The physician complains frequently to the director about Sylvia's work because he feels it goes beyond what a nurse should do. The director meets frequently with Sylvia, trying to solve the problem that exists, although he tells Sylvia that he is in sympathy with her. He tells her she is expected to perform in exactly the manner she has been. Finally, he declares that the problem is merely a "personality conflict" and tells Sylvia to try "being nicer" to the physician.

In this example, Sylvia is caught in the middle. The director is unable to stand up to the physician, and so he vacillates. He functions mainly to transmit the physician's complaints to Sylvia. The problem doesn't get resolved and it's primarily Sylvia who gets hurt.

It probably would have been much better for Sylvia to have confronted the physician and attempted to resolve the problem on her own. Sylvia might have found it effective to network with her colleagues, the social workers, who might have been able to help her understand the behavior of both men in the situation. Although not nurses, they might have had some similar experiences with the physician and psychologist. They might have identified coping behaviors they used in similar situations that Sylvia also could try.

Networking failures also occur when women don't check out situations before they get into them. Take the case of Myrna Coates, an occupational health nurse who accepts a position in a medium-size industry in a neighboring town. The nurse who had worked there previously left rather hastily, but the reasons for her departure remain somewhat of a secret.

Mrs. Coates establishes herself quickly within the Medical Department. She is invited to serve as a member of the Safety Committee, an appointment she eagerly accepts. The committee soon makes recommendations to the Personnel Office; several of the recommendations are Myrna's own. She has devoted much time and energy to these projects. They are complete and well thought out and seem to be enthusiastically endorsed by the committee.

However, Myrna becomes more and more upset as her recommendations are repeatedly rejected by the Personnel Office. She gradually loses interest in her work on the Safety Committee, and increasingly withdraws to the relative safety of the Medical Department. She loses much of her enthusiasm for her job, and contents herself with not trying to make an impact of any kind on the system. She "puts in her eight hours" and goes home.

Some months later, at a meeting of the local chapter of the Occupational Health Nurses' Association, Myrna sees the nurse who previously had worked at the industry where she now works. During their conversation, Myrna learns that the safety officer and the personnel officer have been competing with each other for advancement in the company. Therefore, any suggestions that come from the Safety Committee would probably be rejected by the personnel officer, since if they were good, as Myrna's were, they would help the safety officer rather than the personnel officer advance.

Had Myrna "checked out" with her predecessor before she took the position, she might have been able to avoid appointment to the Safety Committee. On another committee, where such rivalry was not an issue, she would have been able to devote her energies to projects that would have been of more use to the company and more satisfying to her.

Networking also may not work when the women in the network fail to establish a trusting relationship among themselves. In a study of one women's networking group conducted by Carolyn Wysocki and Marc Goldstein, the number of useful contacts made by members did not increase. The authors concluded that ". . . . The exchange of information is, ultimately, based on trust and the expectation of reciprocity. Such feelings and beliefs cannot be created by fiat—the creation of a network does not necessarily create the climate needed to ensure its success."[7]

TRUST IN NETWORKING GROUPS

An essential element in any network is trust. Gibb and Gibb described the four "modal concerns" that differ for those groups that become healthy and productive and those groups that fail. These four concerns are:

- the degree of reciprocal trust among members
- the validity, depth and quality of the feedback system
- the degree of directionality toward group determined goals, and
- the degree of real interdependence in the system.[8]

As described by Gibb and Gibb, trust is the key variable in the growth of any group. If there is not some degree of mutual trust in a group, then members will not be able to communicate with one another. The communications of the group members will be superficial rather than real sharing of feelings, needs, and perceptions.

There are many elements existing in newly formed groups that can be uncomfortable for members. Most often individuals new to a group come together in an environment of uncertainty, anxiety, and distrust. The first concern of the group members is moving toward some certainty and level of comfort.

In an effort to make the situation more comfortable for themselves, group members often perform in predictable ways. Some will try to establish "rules" for the group, in order to provide some form and structure. Others may attempt to force the individuals who originated the group to "take charge" of the group's activities. There is pressure for the group to "do something" and work on tasks is reassuring. The tasks selected generally are "safe" ones that do not involve any personal investment of the members.

At this point, communication is rather polite and formal. Relationships are generally nonpersonal in nature; there is little, if any, self-disclosure. Occasionally, a member may offer some personal information. The result often is that the other members in the group become even more uncomfortable. Many of the members' contributions, whether about feelings or not, are ignored by the group. There is no building on another's communication.

There is a sense of "social distance" among the members. This distance is comforting to those who are anxious about participating in the group. Very little negative feedback is offered, either about a person or the group tasks. At this stage of the group's existence, emotions, particularly anger, are not expressed. Conflict is avoided, although some members may use humor to present negative feelings about the group or what it is doing. It is obvious, then, that at this initial stage of group formation, there is little or no reciprocal trust among the members.

Establishing group goals is a task often attempted by members at this point. Since the members may know very little about one another, they are not aware of one another's goals, particularly those related to joining the group. Therefore, they are unable to work with any degree of efficiency toward group goals that will integrate the goals of the individual members.

Some members of the group may appear most interested and actively involved in the establishment of the group goals. Others may appear almost apathetic, and contribute little to the discussion. Both types are acting as they do because of anxiety about their being in the group. The climate of distrust existing in the group makes them uncomfortable and their behavior patterns reflect their discomfort.

In order for the members to begin to feel more secure in the group, some source of leadership or power must emerge. One person generally "takes charge" and begins to direct the group's work. If more than one person attempts to lead the group, a power struggle occurs. This power struggle, however, is not openly acknowledged. To do so would increase the discomfort of the group members.

In the interim, however, the interdependence of the group members is beginning. As the alliances are established, either "for" or "against" the power source in the group, members start learning to trust one another, first for their own good, and then, increasingly, for the good of the entire group.

As the group progresses, some members will risk sharing feelings. The feelings described generally are those the member had in the past rather than those he or she currently is experiencing. In that way, expressing feelings is made "safer." The feelings often are negative ones that test the group's acceptance, not only of the feeling but of the individual expressing them. These feelings, while negative, usually are couched in positive terms, such as "When I first got in this group, I thought we'd never get anything done because some of the others weren't helping, but we've sure made progress since then!"

If these negative feelings expressed by one of the group members are accepted by the group, then that individual, or someone else, may risk some self-disclosure. Once this phenomenon occurs, it is a sign that trust is beginning in the group. The difference between this self-disclosure and that which may have occurred at the beginning of the group's formation is that in this instance the group pays attention to what is disclosed and in some way deals with the content of the communication.

As trust grows within the group, more and more members are able to offer information about themselves, and the group becomes increasingly accepting. The feedback process gradually becomes more open and honest. The feedback offered helps an individual group member perceive himself or herself as other group members do.

As the group members become more comfortable with individual members' feelings, they are more able to provide support when needed. The humor, seen in earlier stages of the group's development, then used to mask negative feelings about the group, now is used to establish feelings of warmth and closeness among the group members. The humor generally describes "we" situations in the group.

Trust, as it emerges, develops from the positive and negative feelings of the group members. The ability of individuals to express these positive and negative feelings and the ability of the group to accept them are essential elements that must be present if there is to be trust within a group.

BENEFITS OF NETWORKING

In many instances, if nurses had access to information they might have had through networking contacts, they could avoid making costly personal and professional mistakes. Networking takes full advantage of the personal and professional power that results from having access to and using information.

Many acknowledge that information is the power of today. In the past, one's power was largely determined by the amount of land owned. As the nation grew and prospered, power was determined on the basis of personal wealth, or the amount of money you had. In today's times, the most powerful people are not always the richest but those who have access to information.

The information you have access to through your networks can help you advance in your career. You may not know what kind of information you need, but it's what you don't know that can hurt you. You may not even know, at this point, what questions to ask, because you don't know what answers you need. Having access to information will sharpen your skill and ability to sort out information that is useful information, based on your particular needs.

Many successful women attribute their success to "being in the right place at the right time." Explore a bit further and you generally find that these women had access to information that allowed them to move in the right direction at the right time.

Obtaining the right information can assist you in finding employment or in getting promoted in an existing employment situation. Studies have shown that "word of mouth" is a more reliable means for finding employment than the more traditional methods, such as answering want ads or visiting employment agencies.

Information is one of the tangible benefits of networking. Among others are:
- referral
- feedback

Referral

Networking effectively means that you will benefit from referrals. You can be referred to others or you may refer someone who is in your network. When you are referred by someone in your network, you have access to an opportunity that you might not otherwise have had.

Referral through your network carries responsibilities for you. You always must accept the responsibility for whatever task you assume as a result of being referred, so that you do credit not only to yourself but to the individual who referred you. Your behavior as the person referred reflects on the person who referred you.

If you are unable to assume the responsibility, decline gracefully and refer the caller to someone else: "I really can't take on anything more at this time, but I know a bright young nurse who would do an excellent job. Let me get her name and phone number from my file for you."

As an individual in a network, you also have the responsibility to refer others when appropriate. For example, in the following conversation, one individual refers another:

Nurse to editor: I agree, a text on innovative orientation programs for nurses would be useful for the field. That's not my area of expertise, so I am not interested in writing such a text. I do know a young nurse who has been involved in staff development in hospitals for a number of years. She's developed an orientation course that's rather unique. She recently published an article about the program she designed and the article was very well written. Would you be interested in exploring the possibility of writing a book on orientation programs with her? She's here at the conference; I can arrange an introduction and meeting, if you wish.

Or,

Nurse to continuing education director: I've noticed an increased interest in employee performance appraisal here at the hospital. Several of the nurses plan to ask if you would plan a program on that topic. I would like to suggest that you consider asking Allice Meyers to teach the course. She is responsible for the really super performance appraisal process they use at City Hospital. That system is based on job descriptions and standards of nursing practice. She did an impressive job of selling the administration on the changes needed and the nurses there are quite pleased with the way it works. I'd like her to have the opportunity to get some visibility and recognition for her efforts. She's a dynamic speaker. You can contact her at the hospital during the day shift. I have her number here for you.

Thus, the benefits of referral are reciprocal. Members of your network will refer you to professional opportunities and you, in turn, will refer others when opportunities arise that are appropriate and beneficial for them.

Feedback

Feedback is another benefit of networking. Feedback from those with whom you network can help you check out your ideas, even how you dress and other aspects of your behavior, before you actually put anything new into practice. Feedback means there need be little or no risk involved in trying out something new or different for you because you will have checked out the change and confirmed its appropriateness. Those with whom you network can be instrumental in helping you change your current behavior if it's not appropriate for the situations in which you currently must perform.

The feedback you get from others can provide a great psychological lift: "That was a super presentation you gave. Everyone in the audience was so enthusiastic. We can hardly wait to try out those new ideas!"

Feedback can give you a sense of collegiality with other nurses. It's a good feeling to learn that others have similar goals and problems. The effect of knowing that you have colleagues who are experiencing much of what you are generally is a relief to many nurses. It minimizes that feeling of being alone and powerless to do anything about the situations in which you find yourself.

Even if the feedback you receive isn't always positive, it can be helpful. Negative feedback should be offered in a supportive climate, such as that existing in a network, and should be accepted as an attempt to be helpful.

Offering Feedback

Guidelines for giving feedback have been described by Philip G. Hanson, Director of the Human Interaction Training Laboratory at the Houston Veterans' Administration Hospital and noted clinical psychologist and group therapist. Hanson states that it is through feedback that we can learn to "see ourselves as others see us."[9]

Effectively giving and soliciting feedback involves trust, acceptance of others, and the ability to be open in communicating with others, both in sending and receiving messages. Giving feedback is the process that occurs either verbally or nonverbally when an individual lets others know what he or she perceives or thinks about their behavior. When soliciting feedback, an individual asks others to comment on their perceptions and feelings about his or her behavior.

Most people give and receive feedback on an unconscious level. Our reactions to others and theirs to us on a daily basis are feedback of which we may be unaware. But, because this feedback often influences behavior it is important that the feedback be deliberate and conscious in order to be most effective in communicating accurate messages.

One of the most frequent inaccurate messages conveyed to individuals in verbal or nonverbal feedback reflects the confusion between behavior and intentions. People tend to interpret intention from behavior and give feedback on the perceived intention rather than the observed behavior.

For example, an instructor in a continuing education class notices a nurse frowning during the lecture. The instructor immediately responds to the message she perceives the nurse is trying to communicate with her nonverbal behavior by stating "You don't have to agree with what I'm saying; the experts are on my side; I can tell you that I've read a lot in this area and what I'm saying is correct." The instructor here obviously is interpreting the nurse's frown as indicating disagreement. In reality, the nurse may be struggling to understand what the teacher is saying.

It would have been much better for the teacher to offer feedback on the specific observed behavior by saying "You're frowning," and then allow the nurse to interpret her own behavior: "Yes, I'm puzzled . . . I don't understand how that concept fits into the theory discussed earlier."

Giving feedback involves being able to communicate clearly what is meant, so that the individual receiving the feedback understands exactly what was meant and can use the feedback to change his or her behavior. That means the sender of the message must be concerned with the feelings of the person to whom the feedback is being given. The recipient of the feedback must be open and nondefensive when hearing the feedback.

Giving feedback is best accomplished by directly expressing one's feelings. Direct statements of feelings begin with "I" rather than with "you." An individual would say "I am angry with you" rather than "You make me angry," or "I am uncomfortable because you are driving too fast" rather than "You are driving too fast."

Feedback should not be evaluative in nature; that is, the person giving the feedback should not be judging the worth of another person. The feedback should always be in response to a behavior not an individual. For example, an individual can behave stupidly, but that does not mean the person is stupid. In giving feedback in a situation in which a person behaved stupidly, the sender of the message would focus on the stupidity of the behavior rather than on the presumed stupidity of the individual who performed the behavior.

Evaluative feedback offends the person receiving it. In addition, because the feedback is offensive, the individual can't really do anything about changing behavior. Being called "stupid" doesn't help a person know what to change in order to avoid being called stupid again.

Specific feedback is necessary so that the individual knows exactly what response to make. Giving feedback in general terms, such as "You are such an organized person," doesn't let the individual know what behaviors were perceived as organized. More specific feedback would be "I am impressed by the way you organize your daily activities in order of priority."

Feedback should be given immediately after the behavior that provoked it. Delaying feedback, particularly negative feedback, may result in "gunnysacking," that is, dumping a whole sackload of feedback onto a person at one time. In addition to being almost certain to make the person defensive and angry, such a practice often results in the individual having difficulty remembering all his or her past behaviors. The response is likely to be "I don't remember doing [saying] that!"

Feedback may be delayed in an attempt to avoid hurting someone's feelings, or because the person giving the feedback is uncomfortable. If the feedback doesn't immediately follow the behavior, however, it won't be effective.

Feedback should focus on behaviors that a person can change. Many behaviors have become habits, and feedback on these makes the individual uncomfortable. Smoking and overeating are examples of behaviors that are difficult for individuals to change. Calling attention to these behaviors through feedback may only increase the stress of the individual, resulting in even more smoking or overeating. If it seems likely that the behavior can't easily be changed, it would be more appropriate not to offer feedback about that behavior.

Receiving Feedback

When asking for feedback, the same guidelines should be followed. The individual asking for feedback should be specific; for example, "I would like to know how you perceive my ability to speak in public." Asking in general "I would like to know what you think about me" may elicit more information than the individual is prepared to deal with, besides making the person who is responding most uncomfortable.

It is difficult to ask for feedback, because most people are concerned about what they may hear. Asking for feedback implies that there is a trusting relationship. Both individuals involved in a situation where one has asked the other for feedback should be careful not to violate that trust. Since feedback is a reciprocal process, both individuals should help each other in asking for and giving feedback.

Giving feedback is a skill that can be learned and improved upon through practice. Since feedback is an important component of networking, practice in giving feedback also is important to improve one's ability to network. The skilled networker is able to give feedback to others that is helpful and constructive, even if negative.

At the same time, the individual must be comfortable in receiving feedback, recognizing the value of others' perceptions of his or her behavior. If the feedback received isn't helpful, the capable networker will assist the sender of the message to improve his or her ability to give feedback that will be useful.

Networks in which there is caring and trust among the members are a great place in which to give and receive feedback. In such networks, persons can become much more aware of themselves as individuals and can learn how their behavior affects others. These valuable lessons will be of assistance in all their interpersonal relationships, whether within or outside of the network.

NETWORKING CAUTIONS

While networking can do wonders for you, some simple cautions must be considered. The first is that what you get from your network is primarily based on your performance. The networks you participate in won't be helpful to you if you're not already good at what you do. If you don't do good work, for example, another person in your network won't want to refer you for other opportunities for fear that your inability to do well in the new situation will be a poor reflection on him or her.

Another caution is that you must realize that simply participating in a network won't, in and of itself, guarantee instant success. You may get a referral for a job but subsequently not get the job. In your disappointment, you may blame your network. In reality, the reason you didn't get the job could be because you didn't have some of the capabilities the employer was looking for. You may not have had the necessary educational or experiential qualifications. There could be a multitude of other reasons. If you're unable to determine exactly why you didn't get the job, don't take the easy way out and blame the network for failing you. The next referral you get from a member of your network may result in exactly the job you've always wanted.

It is not one of the functions of a network to match individuals with positions. Members of your network can refer you for a job, and can be otherwise helpful in your job search, such as in offering feedback about your resume. But they cannot be held responsible for getting the position you may want for you.

What you get out of your network is directly related to what you put into it. You have to have the basic competencies for your current position and that future position to which you aspire. You have to be responsible for your own professional advancement. Individuals in your networks will be able to assist you, but the primary responsibility is yours. When you recognize and accept these basic cautions about networking, you will be prepared to do it efficiently and effectively.

NETWORKING DOS AND DON'TS

Welch identifies several dos and don'ts both for beginning and more experienced networkers.[10] Among these are:

- do learn how to ask questions
- do try to give as much as you get
- do follow up on contacts
- do keep in touch with your contacts
- do report back to your contacts
- do be businesslike as you network
- don't be afraid to ask for what you need
- don't pass up any opportunities
- don't tell everything to everybody

Asking Questions

Learn how to ask questions when you're networking. Your purpose in asking questions in a networking situation is to get to know the other person. In the process you'll learn how that person may be helpful to you. You want to get as much information from the person as you can, but you also want the individual to get to know you.

Asking effective questions is a skill; it can be learned and improved upon with practice. One way to assess your present level of asking questions is to audio-tape record a conversation during which you are trying to get to know someone, much as you would in a networking situation. Then, you can listen to your cassette recording at your leisure and identify which of the questions you asked were good and which were not.

Good questions are those that elicit information, and give you something on which to base your response. For that reason, questions that elicit a "yes" or "no" answer will be quite limiting for the purposes of further conversation.

For example, compare these questions:

"I liked the speaker tonight, did you?" The response generally will be a "yes" or "no," in which instance, if you want to continue the conversation, you will have to next ask "Why?"

"I thought the speaker tonight was quite provocative. What did you think about him?" In this instance, the individual to whom you are speaking may respond "I thought so too, but he didn't have the same dynamic way of presenting his content as the speaker on the same topic I heard at the nurses' association convention last year." Given this response, you can now pursue (1) further conversation about this speaker, (2) a discussion about the other speaker referred to, or (3) the nurses' association convention.

Questions that do not elicit a "yes" or "no" response are open questions, in contrast to those that close off conversation. In addition to providing you with more information, using open questions will keep you from appearing to be interviewing the individual with whom you wish to converse. Firing a constant stream of questions at someone can be intrusive and defeat your purpose. Then, too, when you run out of questions, the other individual may run out of answers and the conversation will be ended, perhaps even before you've elicited the information you really wanted.

Questions that suggest the answer you want also won't be very helpful in maintaining conversation. For example, when you say "You don't like this workshop, do you?" the person most likely will respond "No," mainly because that's the answer you implied you were expecting. In contrast, asking the individual "How do you like this workshop?" will give you much more information, and you'll learn how the person really feels about the workshop, rather than the way you think he or she feels.

Double-barreled questions have two possible responses from which to choose. Such a question also suggests an answer: "Do you prefer the standard 5-day, 40-hour work week or the 4-day, 10-hour per day work week?" Here the person answering your question has two options for response; you may get an answer but you may never know what kind of work arrangement he or she really prefers. The nurse who asks a co-worker "Are you upset or mad?" may get a response but may not find out that the individual is feeling frustration rather than anger.

Particularly when you're introducing yourself to someone, it's a good idea to include some personal information. You might say "I'm in continuing education for nurses. What do you do?" Or "This is the first time I've been to a national convention. How many have you attended?" Offering some information about yourself is a conversational "tag" that will prove helpful as you continue your discussion.

You also will find useful such conversational "prompts" as "Really?" "Go on . . . ," "Tell me more about that . . . ," or "Describe that further . . ." These prompts encourage the other person to continue talking without your having to ask a question. They also indicate your interest in what the other person is saying. Using prompts can allow you to formulate your response by giving you some extra time to think, but be certain you're not so intent on what you're going to say next that you aren't really listening to the other person. Good listeners are much better conversationalists than those who have the perfect response to every conversational interchange.

Occasionally, you may find yourself the target of a barrage of questions. In that event, try to turn the question back to the other individual. You can say "Yes, I thought the speaker was good. What did you find particularly useful about what she said?"

If the questions are personal, you can reply "No, I've not been divorced. Why would you ask?" Turning these questions back, such as in "No, I've not been divorced. Have you?" will indicate that it's all right to discuss such personal matters but you may not really feel that way. It's best to set limits on personal questions.

If you'd prefer not to respond to a personal question, simply say "Why would you ask that question?" If you answer without anger in your voice the person asking the question should get the message that personal questions are off limits and refrain from asking any more.

Be sure that your questions do not invade another person's privacy. If a personal question of another individual is important to your conversation, preface it with information on the same topic about yourself. Saying "I felt really upset when I was turned down for that position. Have you ever experienced a similar situation?" is less uncomfortable for the person from whom you expect a response than "Have you ever been turned down for a job you wanted?"

Giving Help

Helping others in your networks is as important as being helped. Try to be as helpful as possible to others. It may not be enough to demonstrate your willingness to help through your nonverbal behavior. You may have to offer to help in verbal terms.

Your offer of assistance will be more useful if it is specific than if it is general. For example, "If you have any problems with the evaluation, let me know" is not as specific as "When it's time for analysis of the evaluative data, I'll be glad to help."

Assistance with problematic personal and professional situations is one of the major benefits of networking. It may well be that you help others from whom you do not get any assistance. In turn, others help you and you may not necessarily return their assistance. Nonetheless, the benefits of your networking are reciprocal, since you are helping and being helped in exchange. Without any such exchange of assistance, networks would collapse, and women would stop helping women.

Following Up

When you offer your help, it is imperative that you follow through. If you make a promise to provide information or a referral, be sure you do it. You may have to devise a way of keeping track of what you say you'll do so that you remember and can do it. For some people, always carrying a note pad and pencil and writing down follow-up actions has been the most effective way for them to keep track. Others commit their necessary networking follow-up activities to memory. Use whatever works best for you to ensure that you do what you say you will.

When others offer their help to you, accept willingly. If their help is not needed, decline graciously. Try not to decline help because you don't want to be a nuisance or bother to anyone. If help is offered, assume it is offered freely.

If someone suggests other individuals whom you should know, be certain you follow up on the suggestion. Make the acquaintance of the individuals suggested and then report the results of your meeting to the person who made the original suggestion. In addition to being an excellent way of expanding your network, you are providing information to your contact about the success of his or her referrals.

Keeping in Touch

Keep in touch with members of your network. Occasional telephone calls are all that is necessary to let them know you are thinking about them. These phone calls can be made for "no reason at all" except to see how an individual is doing. Calling only when you want something sets up the situation where the person being called thinks, when hearing you're on the other end of the line, "Oh, no, now what does she want?"

You may be more comfortable writing occasional notes to those in your networks to keep in touch. Enclosing a newspaper clipping of interest to an individual adds a personal touch. Sending post cards from conference or convention sites also lets members of your network know you're thinking of them.

Keep in touch with former co-workers and others even if they no longer are members of your current network. An effective networker never burns bridges. Some of the best future opportunities arise from previous contacts.

Reporting Back

If someone refers you for a job, an interview, or any other professional opportunity, report back. Send a simple thank-you note, or make a brief phone call to convey your appreciation for the assistance. This is common courtesy and is meaningful to your contact. Besides, your contact will remain interested in your progress. Knowing you appreciate the referral may make it more likely that you will be referred again in the future. Reporting back is an excellent way of maintaining a relationship with your contacts.

If possible, notify a contact when you've made a referral to him or her. Even better is to call and confirm that making the referral is all right with the individual. Either way you're using another means of keeping in touch with your contacts.

Being Businesslike

Be businesslike in your relationships with contacts. The primary purpose of networking is to help you get ahead in your profession, not to meet your social needs. Brief telephone conversations about items of interest to members of your network should suffice. It may be better in some instances to communicate with particularly busy contacts in writing. That way the individual can respond to you at his or her convenience. Communicating in writing rather than by telephone will prevent your interrupting a busy individual at work, or, worse yet, having your call screened by a secretary who won't let you interrupt the busy boss.

Avoid the tendency to bring into your networking relationships much that is personal in your life. While the individuals with whom you network may be interested in hearing about your spouse and children, the primary purpose of networking is professional. You may not be confronted about this breach of the networking "rules," but, nonetheless, your future networking efforts may suffer because you obviously don't know how to play the game.

Asking for Help

Don't be afraid to ask for what you want from members of your network. If no one knows what you want, no one can help you get it. If an individual in your network is unable (or unwilling) to assist you, assume that you will be told so by the person himself or herself. If you aren't told, then assume that the assistance you asked for is being provided willingly.

As you seek assistance from members of your network, avoid seeking out only one individual for everything you need. You can place too much of a burden on that one person. There probably are others in the network who would be willing, and just as able, to help if you asked them.

Also be certain you're well prepared before you ask for assistance. Read up on the topic before asking questions, particularly of "experts" in the area.

Ask questions that are specific rather than general. Don't ask someone to tell you all he or she knows about continuing education, for instance. Read up on the subject so that your question is focused, such as "What have been the experiences of states with continuing education requirements for relicensure in relation to increased costs of the license renewal process?''

Don't be afraid to approach someone who is well-known for assistance. Do, however, use common sense in your approach to such a person. When you meet, write, or call the person, state the nature of your business briefly and concisely. Don't ask for or expect help that will take a large amount of time. Ask for reasonable assistance, and give the person an opportunity to graciously refuse.

Don't be afraid to approach someone whom you perceive to be a very "busy" person. You may think that such a busy person won't have time for you. However, the busiest people often are the ones who are most willing to take the time to help when needed.

Again, in this instance as in many others, the benefits of networking are reciprocal. On the one hand, you are getting help from someone "famous"; and, on the other hand, you are giving that person the satisfaction of knowing that he or she was helpful to you. Moreover, "famous" people like to know what's going on, to keep in touch, and assume roles of leadership.

When you ask for assistance, and it's offered, be careful what you do next. If you expect an answer to all of your problems, you surely will be disappointed. There are few, if any, "instant" problem solutions, even in the most effective networks. Ultimately, the problem is your responsibility, as is the solution to that problem. Persons in your networks can offer advice and support to you as you work through the problem, but they can't solve it for you.

It may be that the best response to your problem that you receive from your network is that others listen to you. Talking about a problem with a sympathetic listener gives us the opportunity to clarify our own thinking and to "hear" how the problem sounds to others. Often, just getting the problem out into the open is helpful.

If, in the course of a conversation about a problem for which you are seeking assistance, someone proposes a solution, accept the advice in the spirit of helpfulness in which it was offered. Remember, the final decision about whether to follow through on the advice or reject it is yours. It is better that you make that final decision when you're alone, not in the company of the person who offered the advice, particularly if you are rejecting it. It is frustrating to those who are trying to help you to hear responses such as "I've already tried that," "That won't work for me," or "I could do that, but. . . ."

Using Opportunities

Be absolutely sure that you take advantage of every opportunity to network. Any time you are in a situation with members of your network, or with those individuals whom you wish to add to your network, is an appropriate time to network.

Although the purpose of networking is primarily for your professional advancement, don't neglect networking with women who are in more traditional positions, such as homemakers. These women also have contacts in their own various networks that can be most useful to you.

Include in your networks people of all ages. While some may have little in common with you at one point in time, there may be a time when you share interests. Learning from others who have been there is most helpful. Learning can take place even from the inexperienced, for creativity has no age requirements. And the young are often "where the action is."

Even events that seem primarily social, like meals and parties, are good occasions on which to network. Much that is important and helpful to you can be accomplished in such a relaxed atmosphere. Much of men's networking occurs in exactly these types of away-from-work situations.

When at a party or other social situation, circulate as much as possible among the guests. You never know when you will meet a valuable contact. Begin meeting these new contacts by introducing yourself. Comments about the party or other event you are attending will help "break the ice."

Remember that most people like to talk about themselves, so direct your questions and comments toward conversation about the other person rather than yourself. If you are uncomfortable about meeting other people, try to set goals for yourself, so that at the first event you meet three new people, then five, then eight, and so on. As you practice meeting new individuals, it will become easier and less uncomfortable.

While you're moving around meeting new people, don't neglect those you already know. Try to say something to everyone in the room whom you know. Do, however, enjoy the event you're attending. While you want to keep in touch with previous contacts and make new ones, your primary purpose should be to attend the event, whether a meeting or a social occasion. Your focus should not be exclusively on networking, but networking can be a benefit derived from many situations in which you find yourself.

As you are networking in social rather than business situations, be sensitive to others' need to get away from business to relax. Timing is important, whether you are networking in business or social situations. If your contact isn't responding as enthusiastically to your networking efforts as you might wish, it may be better to make an appointment for another time when both of you would be at the same point in relation to the purpose for your meeting.

When you're traveling, use the opportunity to network with individuals in the cities to which you go. If you don't know anyone in a particular city, perhaps someone else in your network does and can refer you to people who live in that city. In this way, you will expand your contacts outside of your immediate geographic area, and will have colleagues with whom to socialize while in an unfamiliar place. These contacts are useful for providing information such as the best local hairdresser, restaurants, hotels, theaters, and so on to make your stay in a city away from home more pleasant.

Take advantage of every opportunity to keep expanding your networks, both in your home town and elsewhere. You never know when or where you will need a contact.

Being Discreet

Information is a critical component of networking. For some members of a particular network, information may be the primary benefit. You may have information that is of use to others in your network, especially if you know something before it's general knowledge. Be certain that by telling something you're not betraying a confidence. Otherwise, your reputation will suffer, and, perhaps more important for your networking efforts, you may not be given such "advance notice" information again.

Be careful about telling all the "gory details," particularly if the story involves others. You may be quite interested in referring a colleague for a job, and, in your eagerness, tell all you know about your friend. The prospective employer does not need to know, for example, that she recently was divorced and is having difficulty adjusting to single-parent status. If your colleague wishes to relate that information, that is her decision, but such personal and not job-related information should not come from you.

Be cautious, also, about revealing too much information about yourself. Women are particularly prone to reveal negative aspects about themselves. Networking involves communicating positive aspects about ourselves; negative topics of conversation should be the exception rather than the rule.

Again, networking should be primarily businesslike in nature. Only personal information that directly affects that business is appropriate for inclusion in your networking efforts. All other personal information, about yourself or others, is irrelevant.

Finally, although you may have successful attempts at networking, don't be discouraged if not every effort is successful. If you let one, or even several, failures convince you that networking is not for you, you will be doing yourself a disfavor.

Sometimes events beyond our control influence the success of a networking try. You may be able to pick up clues about what went wrong by reviewing the networking attempt. It could be that the person you approached was too busy, or just had been asked by several others for favors, or a myriad of other reasons. If, as you review the incident in your mind, you become aware that the person left the door open, try the networking approach again.

If the incident seemed to result in a closed door for you, review what you said and did as well as what the other person said and did. You may be able to get some notion about where the negative reaction began by reviewing the entire conversation. Perhaps you missed a cue that this was not a good time to ask for something. If the other person said "What a day; just when I think I have myself together, some other thing comes up. It never ends!" and you pursued your original intent and asked for a favor, almost surely the result would be a negative response.

It also may be helpful to review the incident with other members of your network. They may be able to offer feedback on your networking effort that you are not able to view as objectively. If possible, role play the incident, so that you convey the incident as clearly and accurately as possible. In the role play, it will be more helpful if you play the part of the other individual. Someone else should play your part; you will need to coach that person about your behavior, verbal and nonverbal, during the incident. This more objective review of the networking failure may provide feedback about changes in your behavior in future networking attempts.

SUMMARY

You may experience an initial excitement about your networking efforts, particularly if they go well. Then you may find that things don't go as well as they initially did. While it is thrilling to have networking efforts really work for us, networking does not always work. When networking efforts are successful, they are not necessarily consistently successful, that is, networking does not happen every time it is attempted.

Often, also, the results of our networking efforts are not immediately apparent. It may be months or years before something occurs as a result of a previous networking attempt.

The excitement of networking is sustained, however, when you begin to realize how helpful networks are in assisting you to meet your professional goals. When you discover that you have colleagues who are genuinely concerned about you and what you want, and, further, who take pleasure in helping you get what you want, you will experience the joy of networking.

NOTES

1. Carol Kleinman, *Women's Networks* (New York: Ballantine Books, 1980), pp. 207–287.

2. Mary Scott Welch, *Networking* (New York: Harcourt Brace Jovanovich, 1980), p. 15.

3. E. L. Shostrom, *Man, the Manipulator* (New York: Abingdon Press, 1967), p. 15.

4. Kleinman, *Women's Networks*, p. 4.

5. "Equitable Employees Create Communication Networks," Life Office Management Association, *Resource*, July/August, 1978, pp. 12–13.

6. "Organizing Women at the Top," *Time*, April 19, 1982, p. 65.

7. Marc B. Goldstein and Carolyn M. Wysocki, "Is Networking Working? A Case Study of a Women's Network," mimeographed (New Britain: Central Connecticut State College, 1982).

8. Jack R. Gibb and Lorraine M. Gibb, "Humanistic Elements in Group Growth," *Challenges of Humanistic Psychology* (New York: McGraw-Hill, 1967), pp. 161–170.

9. Phillip G. Hanson, "Giving Feedback: An Interpersonal Skill," *The 1975 Annual Handbook for Group Facilitators* (La Jolla, Calif.: University Associates), pp. 147–154.

10. Welch, *Networking*, pp. 98–111.

Chapter 2

How To Use Networking

Once you've decided to use networking to get what you what, you will want to use your networking skills as effectively and efficiently as possible. Networking well takes time and effort, but the results make the expenditure of time and effort worthwhile.

We've all heard and read about "coupon clippers," people who cut and save "cents off" coupons for grocery purchases as well as redeem coupons for special offers or refunds. Individuals who devote time to organizing a system for saving and redeeming coupons report results that are far more lucrative than the efforts of those of us who participate more haphazardly.

So it is with networking. It does require time and energy to network. The initial time required to assess one's networks and decide whether to expand them, as well as the time needed to organize those networks, ultimately pays off with career advancement opportunities that may have otherwise not existed for us.

While there are many "how-to" books for women on the market, there has been little written that will assist women who wish to advance their careers. Magazines that are devoted to such issues often are looked upon as too feminist—too radical—too strident in their call for change in the working world to make it more accommodating to women. What often happens is information that is of value to the reader is overlooked because of a superficial review of the magazine's contents. Similarly, the value of networking as a technique should not be overlooked by the nurse seeking some change in his or her personal and professional life.

The existing literature on networking encourages women initially to realize that they "can't make it alone." In support of this idea, much of the content of networking books and articles is devoted to trying to overcome the stereotype of women not getting along with each other and of women instinctively mistrusting other women. Part of the reason for this stereotype stems from the mistaken notion that other women are not to

31

be trusted with one's male friends. Although networking can be used in your personal life (and may ultimately involve relationships with men), the primary purpose of networking is to assist in advancing your professional career. In this context, women can serve a useful purpose for you rather than being your competition.

Nurses, by and large, aren't victims of that unflattering stereotypical thinking about other women. Most nurses realize from the beginning of their professional lives that they are members of the health care team, and that they must work with one another for the ultimate benefit of the patient. Many members of the health care team other than nurses also are women, so women working with women in the context of delivering health care services is generally the norm in the nursing profession. While not all of these relationships are characterized by harmony, neither are other interpersonal relationships, regardless of the sex of the participants.

Nurses, therefore, can begin the process of networking without the interference of such stereotypes about their relationships with other women. Using networking effectively and enthusiastically also will have as a potential side benefit helping to eliminate such stereotypical thinking on the part of others.

PREPARING TO NETWORK

Once you've decided to network to get what you want for yourself professionally, there is some advance preparation necessary. In order to network effectively you have to possess the "tools of the trade." You will want to be able to make the best use of your time in order to be able to allocate time for important networking activities.

Among the other necessary elements for effective networking are that you have a well-prepared curriculum vitae or resume, and that you present yourself well. An important component of presenting yourself well is how you look. How you look is influenced by how you dress, your hairstyle, and your makeup.

Of course, this is not to say that your professional success will depend only on what you wear: "Clothing does not make the woman." In order to attain your professional goals you will need to be competent in your area of practice, possess reasonable intelligence, and be ambitious enough to want to move up the ladder of success in the nursing profession.

MANAGING YOUR TIME

Most nurses don't have unlimited time to spend on career advancement. There are other obligations that often take priority—home and family, for instance. If networking is to be helpful in meeting your professional goals, you must spend time on networking activities. In order to do that, you may have to eliminate some other activities. Time management is a process that helps you eliminate activities in your life that are least important so that you can concentrate on those activities that are most important.

In order to use the time management process, you must ask yourself these questions:

- What do I want to accomplish?
- How am I organizing my activities to accomplish what I want to?
- What results am I having in relation to what I want to accomplish?[1]

Your responses to these questions will provide you with an idea about the activities in which you currently are engaged.

Another way of assessing your current activities is to keep a daily log for a least a week and preferably two. Log your activities on a 15-30 minute basis. Include in this log the time you start an activity, the time it ends, what the activity was, who was involved in the activity, who initiated the activity, and what the end result of the activity was. Keep this log for both your professional and your personal time. You may find that the only real time you have to devote to networking activities is time after your work.[2]

Once you've determined how you spend your time, you can learn to practice some of the many time management techniques in order to more effectively use your time. Among the most successful of these time management techniques are:

- plan your daily activities, both professional and personal
- put your daily plan in writing
- prioritize things you have to do
- do the most important activities first
- combine activities whenever possible
- check off activities as they're completed
- review the list of daily activities frequently to keep on-target
- do not over-schedule your work day
- avoid interruptions
- organize your work setting for maximum efficiency
- delegate any task that can be delegated
- learn to say "no"
- process paperwork faster by only handling a piece of paper once; deal with it the first time you handle it

- do only one thing at a time
- leave undone those activities with the lowest priority
- take your scheduled breaks and meal periods
- periodically evaluate how you are using your time.[3]

THE CURRICULUM VITAE

Another essential element in your preparation for networking is having a well-prepared curriculum vitae.[4] A curriculum vitae (plural curricula vitae) is defined by the *Random House Collegiate Dictionary* as "the course of one's life or career." A curriculum vitae generally is contrasted with a resume, which is a chronological account of your life's experiences, primarily used to obtain an interview for a desired position.

The curriculum vitae, or CV, is usually designed for the purpose of presenting educational and experiential qualifications (see Exhibit 2-1). Thus, the CV can be used in various situations, such as when you are seeking employment or being introduced as a speaker.

A CV has two important elements: appearance and currency. It reflects your professional and/or personal achievements. It should be carefully prepared. It is a good idea to make an outline of the information you wish to include in your CV before beginning to type. In this way you can review the information before the CV is finalized to assure yourself that irrelevant information is not being included.

The CV should be professionally typed and should not contain errors, such as strike-overs or misspelled words. Avoid adding information using different typewriter elements, or, worse yet, handwriting. The CV you provide to others need not be an original copy; photocopies are acceptable. The CV should be copied onto good quality bond paper and should be a "clean" copy. Many of the instant print shops will photocopy your CV adequately. You will want enough copies for immediate use, but not so many that when activities need to be added you discard large quantities.

Many of us prepared our first CV by copying someone else's. This practice perpetuates errors in the appropriate preparation of a CV. A CV is more structured than a resume, and so fewer liberties should be taken in its preparation.

Information to be placed on a CV includes:

- name, title, address, and telephone number
- social security number (optional)
- post-secondary education

Exhibit 2–1

CURRICULUM VITAE

NAME: Zimmerman, Nancy Joan

HOME ADDRESS: 2019 65th Street, Apt 201A
                         New York, New York 10023
                         Telephone: (098) 123-4567

BUSINESS ADDRESS: Mount Mary College
                         Department of Nursing
                         2000 West Drive
                         New York, New York 00123
                         Telephone: (098) 765-4321

EDUCATION:

Degrees	Degree Granting Institution	Preparation	Year
Ph.D.	University of New York New York, New York	Nursing	1981
M.S.N.	University of New York New York, New York	Nursing	1979
B.S.N.	University of New York New York, New York	Nursing	1976

EXPERIENCE:

1981 to
present   Professor, Graduate Department
                 Medical-Surgical Nursing
                 Mount Mary College
                 New York, New York

1979 to
1981   Associate Professor, Graduate Department
                 Medical-Surgical Nursing
                 Mount Mary College
                 New York, New York

1978 to
1979   Assistant Professor, Graduate Department
                 Medical-Surgical Nursing
                 Mount Mary College
                 New York, New York

1976 to
1978   Instructor, Undergraduate Program
                 Medical-Surgical Nursing
                 Mount Mary College
                 New York, New York

Exhibit 2–1 continued

RESEARCH:

Zimmerman, Nancy Joan. *Pain Management Through Biofeedback.* Unpublished doctoral dissertation, University of New York, N.Y., 1981.

_____. *Medical-Surgical Approaches to Pain Management.* Unpublished master's thesis, University of New York, N.Y., 1979.

PROFESSIONAL ACTIVITIES:

American Nurses' Association
Sigma Theta Tau
Who's Who in American Nurses
Society for Research on Pain Management

PUBLICATIONS:

Zimmerman, Nancy Joan, "Pain and the Medical–Surgical Nurse," *American Journal of Nursing,* 1982, *74,* 2013–2019.

_____, "Nurses' Responsibility for Pain Control" in *Nurses' Role in Health Care,* Margaret Murray (Ed), New York, N.Y.: Smith Publishing Co., 1980.

- work experience
- honors
- research completed or ongoing
- grants or awards received
- professional organization activities
- publications

Include with your name your employer's name and business address. If your preferred mailing address is your home, indicate that. The telephone number on your CV should be one at which you can easily be reached during regular business hours. If you are not available during those times, indicate some usual times when you can be reached. Be certain that zip codes are included with addresses and area codes are included with telephone numbers.

Do not list your academic credentials after your name; those will be apparent on review of the section on education. Do not include information on your CV about your marital status, number of children, state of health, and so on.

Your social security number is an optional entry on your CV. However, if you are being paid for consulting, teaching, or lecturing, your social security number will be necessary for reporting that income to the Internal

Revenue Service. Having your social security number on your CV may prevent someone from having to make an additional contact with you to obtain the number.

Education

In reverse chronological order, from the most to the least recent, list your post-secondary educational experiences. In this listing include (1) the institution, (2) the location, (3) the degree received and when, and (4) the field of study. If the degree is commonly known, abbreviations are adequate. If the degree is not a common one, spell it out. If you are certified, include the specifics in this section.

You may wish to include a subsection here for continuing education attendance. It is imperative that you be selective about what continuing education activities you choose to include. Only those of scholarly merit should be entered. If you are preparing your CV for a specific audience, for example, to teach a continuing education activity on a specific topic, include your attendance at relevant continuing education activities.

Include degrees you expect to receive only if you are close to receiving them. Exercise caution in using the terms "doctoral student" and "doctoral candidate" interchangeably; they have different meanings. A doctoral student is one who has been accepted into a doctoral program and who is currently involved in course work. A doctoral candidate is one who generally has completed course work (or very nearly so) and also has passed the qualifying examinations for admission into candidacy. While such an error is innocently made in most instances, if you make the error on your CV, you may be viewed as deliberately misrepresenting yourself.

Experience

The section on work experience should include all of your professional employment. List these in reverse chronological order, including (1) dates of employment, (2) position title, (3) agency, and (4) location.

If the position title is not a common one, you can insert a descriptor that is more commonly understood. For example, if you are listing a position such as "Patient Care Coordinator," you may insert in parentheses "(Supervisor)." Be certain to include the area of practice in which you were employed, such as "orthopedic nursing," "psychiatric/mental health nursing," and so on.

The section on research completed or ongoing should include your master's thesis and/or doctoral dissertation. Any research projects that you have completed or in which you currently are involved, in addition to master's and doctoral studies, should be included here.

If you've participated in any funded project, either as an individual or as part of a group, include the specifics in this section. Describe those projects with which you were involved either in the grant-writing stage, as an investigator, or directing in any capacity. If a project was approved but not subsequently funded, it is appropriate to include it. However, do not list projects that were not approved for funding.

In the "honors" section, include honors that you have been awarded, such as commencement honors (degrees awarded cum laude, or summa cum laude). Memberships in such organizations as Sigma Theta Tau, the national nurses' honorary society, or Phi Beta Kappa are appropriate for inclusion here.

Professional Activities

In the section on professional activities, list current memberships in organizations related to your professional life. Only current memberships should be included. Also include any offices held in these organizations, and the dates you were in office, either elected or appointed. Include committee service. It is not appropriate for a CV to contain your memberships in social or civic organizations.

Professional activities other than memberships should be included in a subsection. Describe any activities such as consultations, serving on students' thesis or dissertation committees, teaching in continuing education programs, and the like. Exercise selectivity about what you include here lest you give the appearance of "padding" your CV.

Publications

Finally, your CV should contain a listing of your publications. Follow a style guide when listing publications in this section in order to be certain that references to your publications are complete, consistent, and appropriately punctuated. This listing also should be in reverse chronological order.

If there was more than one author on a publication, list the senior author first. Publications that have not yet appeared in print should be listed as "in press." If you are aware of the estimated date of publication, include that date with your citation.

It is important to be selective in what you include in this section. A general rule of thumb is to include only those publications that appeared in major, national print media. Presentations in "Proceedings of Conferences" are acceptable, but preferably they should be invited scholarly papers. A paper you submitted in response to a "Call for Papers," which was chosen for presentation through blind review (a process by which papers are reviewed and selected without the reviewers knowing the name of the individual submitting the paper), also is acceptable for inclusion in this section.

It generally is not appropriate to include your contributions to primarily local publications, such as the newsletter of a professional association. A guideline here is that the publication should not be included if it is part of your job. For example, if you are president of a professional nursing association's local or state chapter, and it is "part of your job" to write a "Call to Convention" or to contribute a column to the association's newsletter on a periodic basis, you would not include those "publications" in this section.

Instead list this as an activity in the "Professional Activities" subsection of your CV. There you can list your presidency under offices held, and include a reference such as "contributed 'President's Column' monthly to the association newsletter."

Similarly, if you are the editor of a newsletter and that is part of your job, the position of editor should be included in the section on your professional experiences rather than in the publications section. If not a significant contribution to the nursing (or related) literature, it is better to omit a reference than to have your CV appear "hyped up." If you have doubts about what publications could be omitted, you may wish to seek advice from an individual who has published extensively.

In order to indicate clearly to the reader of your CV that you did exercise discretion in listing professional activities and publications, you may wish to title those sections "Selected Professional Activities" and "Selected Publications." This notation says without a doubt that there were other entries you chose not to include. Be certain, however, that publications that are omitted are not those, for example, that earned criticism in a book review or a letter to the editor. Your CV should reflect the best of your professional efforts, but dishonesty is not acceptable.

Finally, your CV should be dated. The CV should be updated whenever significant additions or changes occur. The person who types your CV often can arrange spacing so that there is room for additions without having to retype the complete CV because of an additional consultation, presentation, or publication.

THE RESUME

A resume is a document that is designed to advertise who you are in terms of what you are competent to do, what you have accomplished in

Exhibit 2–2 Sample Resume

	RESUME	
	MARY LYNN WEAVER	
439 Center Street	Center City, Iowa	123/456-7890

OBJECTIVE:	A clinical specialist position . . . leading to administration . . . of a mental health clinic where my interpersonal, administrative, and therapeutic skills will be used for the advancement of mental health care for citizens of the state.
EMPLOYMENT EXPERIENCES:	1980–present Supervised establishment of inpatient psychiatric unit in general hospital. Memorial Hospital, Center City, Iowa. Provided consultation to community mental health nurses' organization, Center City, Iowa.
	1977–1980 (part-time) Clinical Counselor Worked as staff nurse in Corner Clinic in alcohol and addiction program.
EDUCATION:	*M.S. in Nursing,* 1980 University of Iowa, Center City, Iowa.
	B.S. in Nursing, 1977 University of Iowa, Center City, Iowa.
PERSONAL:	32 . . . excellent health . . . single . . . member of American Nurses' Association, Clinical Counselors of America.
REFERENCES:	Available upon request.

the past, and what you are capable of doing in the future (see Exhibit 2-2). A resume has as its primary purpose helping you get interviews, which will lead to job offers.

An effective resume combines the elements of form and content. Neither should be emphasized at the expense of the other. The form of your resume is what will attract the attention of the prospective employer. The resume should be pleasant in appearance and easy to read. Resumes with a poor layout, or that contain typographical errors, misspellings, bad grammar, incorrect punctuation, or that are poorly typed or duplicated contain serious flaws. These errors in resume form may determine whether you will be invited for an interview.

Errors in the substance of the resume also influence your chances of getting an interview. If the resume doesn't accurately reflect your accomplishments, if there isn't sufficient content, if there are unexplained gaps in time between jobs, or if it appears you are boasting or dishonest, the content of the resume will fail to communicate your professional objectives, abilities, and experience.

A resume is developed through a three-stage process, as described by Krannich and Banis, authors of *High Impact Resumes & Letters.*[5] They describe the three steps as:

- preparation
- writing
- production

Preparing the Resume

Krannich and Banis recommend that individuals prepare their own resumes.[6] There are commercial services that will prepare resumes for a reasonable fee, but these services often use a standardized format that may not reflect an individual's unique capabilities.

Although the preparation stage is initially time consuming, the time is well spent if the resume accomplishes its purpose. As updates of the resume are needed, only minimal time will be required if the resume is initially well constructed.

The first information on your resume should be how to contact you. Include here your name, address, and telephone number. Include zip codes with addresses and area codes with telephone numbers. This information should be eye catching and well placed at the top of the resume.

The next information on your resume should be your professional objective. This should be a concise statement of what you want to do and what you have to offer a prospective employer. The position you are seeking is what you want to do, and your educational and experiential background is what you have to offer. This objective should be position- or job-oriented rather than self-oriented, that is, the objective should reflect what you have to offer rather than emphasize what you want out of a job.

The process to be used to identify your professional objective is described in many of the texts available on writing resumes. Krannich and Banis describe four steps in the objective development process:

- obtain data on your skills,

- corroborate this data with information from others and from yourself, through a series of exercises,
- project your preferences into the future, again through a series of exercises, and
- test your objective against reality.[7]

A professional objective should be composed of a general statement of your skills and the proposed outcome of the application of those skills. For example, the statement of your objective could read "I would prefer a job where I can use my ability to. . . . . .which will result in. . . . . . ."[8]

The objective statement should be specific enough so that the prospective employer immediately understands what you want and what you have to offer. The objective should be written with a particular position in mind; this will aid in writing an objective that is as specific as possible.

Next on the resume should appear a description of your past experiences. Describe all of your past professional experiences in terms of what you actually did. Use active verbs to describe your accomplishments. Use words like: "coordinated," "planned," "implemented," "supervised," "initiated," and so on.

Experiences should be listed in reverse chronological order. List dates of employment first, followed by the job title and description of your responsibilities. End with the employer's name and address.

The section on your educational background can be situated either before or after your experiences, depending on the emphasis you wish to place on it. List education in reverse chronological order. If there were specific additional achievements in your educational endeavors, list those immediately below the education statement that indicates the degree obtained, location of the college/university, and date.

A sample statement of such achievements is:

> Ph.D. in Higher Education, University of Indiana, Indianapolis, 1981. Related courses include Statistics, Research, Business Administration. Maintained a Q.P.A. of 4.7 (5.0 index).

Educational accomplishments can be stated without additional information. These statements would read:

> Ph.D. in Higher Education, University of Indiana, Indianapolis, 1981.
> M.S. in Business Administration, University of Ohio, Cleveland, 1977.

If you have educational accomplishments in addition to your academic degrees, a section titled "Additional Education" can be added to your resume. Include in this section information on diplomas or certification you have received.

Next on your resume should be a section on personal information. Include a statement that describes you as an individual. You can note hobbies, special interests, or abilities that distinguish you from other applicants whose resumes also will be read. This personal statement should relate as much as possible to your professional objective.

Avoid including information in this section about personal characteristics such as height, weight, state of your health, marital status, number of children, and so on, unless you are certain these characteristics will be looked upon favorably by the prospective employer. If you are not certain that it is essential to include this information, it is better omitted.

The next section on a resume should relate to your personal references. Because you may choose different individuals as references for different positions, indicate in this section that references are available upon request. Have available when you go for an interview a typed list of individuals who will provide a reference for you. (It is common courtesy to request permission to list an individual as a reference before you do so.) List the individual's name, title, employer, address, and telephone number.

You also may wish to include on your resume such miscellaneous categories as professional memberships and activities, licensure, and available date of employment. Include other information only as it is related to your professional objective.

Writing the Resume

You probably will need to write several drafts of your resume. Begin by listing all of the information you've collected on your experiences and education. Review what you've written to be certain it relates to what you said was your professional objective. Review what you've written a second time to be certain it's clear and concise and expresses exactly what you want to say.

Have several colleagues review the drafts of your resume and offer suggestions for improvement. If possible, have an individual who is responsible for hiring review the resume. Such a person should have seen a variety of resumes and so can effectively critique yours.

Your resume should not be over two pages in length, and preferably only one. If there is more information on the resume than can be accommodated in two pages, it would be wise to eliminate sections such as

"Personal Information" or "References" to reduce the length of the document.

Producing the Resume

Have your resume professionally typed. The layout of the resume is important for its eye appeal. Use "white space" to set off the various sections and to enhance readability.

Use quality bond paper for the original copy and for the copies you have duplicated. Duplicate only the number of copies you estimate you will use in the near future. All of the copies should be perfect; those copies with streaks, tracks, or smudges should be destroyed.

Use white paper or a pale shade of gray, beige, or off-white. Ink color can be other than black but should complement the chosen paper color. Avoid extremes of color either in the paper or the ink.

DRESSING FOR SUCCESS

The physical aspects of preparing yourself for networking include dressing for success. As more and more nurses are moving away from having to wear uniforms at work, clothes become a more crucial item in a nurse's professional life. Nurses, however, most will say, don't generally earn salaries large enough to afford the kind of clothes they need to dress as "fashion plates" for work. Most people who have time to shop and unlimited funds to shop with often end up with the same problem: they just have larger closets filled with "nothing to wear."

Clothes You Have

A bit of organized effort may well solve the clothes problem. A first step is self-analysis. Look at the clothes you are now wearing. Try everything on in good light, in front of a full-length mirror, preferably one that allows you simultaneously to get side views. If you don't have such a mirror, use a hand mirror to get side and back views. Try on all of your clothes, looking specifically at such things as color, fit around the waist, bust, and hips, hemlines, and necklines.

Look next at what kind of clothes are suitable for your life style. If you work in street clothes rather than in a uniform, the clothes you wear must be suitable for your work and the environment in which you work.

Look next at the mix and match of your existing wardrobe. Hang your clothes in the closet by types—jackets together, skirts together, pants together, and blouses together. That way you'll get beyond seeing only coordinates purchased together as matches. Experiment a bit! Use individuals in your network to give you feedback on your various outfits; but get a variety of opinions before you finally decide either positively or negatively about an outfit since individual tastes vary.

Another type of feedback that is useful when you are dressing to get ahead is that which you get spontaneously. What outfits are you wearing on which you are often complimented? What makes you feel terrific when you wear it?

All of this information is useful when preparing your wardrobe. Once you have a firm notion of what you now have, you can begin to decide what else you need. Start by visiting local stores to try on clothes. The key here is "trying on"; you're not at the buying stage yet. Spend lots of time trying on clothes of different styles, fabrics, and colors. Go to the best stores and to the best departments in them. You always can find bargains or sales later when you're actually ready to buy. Start at the top with your trying on stage; the clothes are generally made better and fit better.

Even if you think it can't possibly look good on you, try it on anyway. You're trying here to get an idea of what does look best on you, so you must try on a large variety of items to pin down the few best. Of all the variety of items you try on, you will find some that always look good on you. Many will be marginal in their appearance and some will look absolutely awful—better to have left them on the hanger.

The key here is to remember what always looks good on you—what colors, what styles, what lengths, and what fabrics. It is important, too, to be aware that what you might want to look good on you may not.

It is equally important that you go alone to do your trying on. This is not the time for feedback from your friends, even your closest and dearest ones. You need to see your wardrobe primarily through your own eyes rather than through theirs. If, when you are wearing an outfit you've selected because it looks so good on you, your friends' feedback is overwhelmingly positive, you'll know you've succeeded in selecting clothes that are you.

Clothes You Need

Now that you've tried on clothes and have learned what looks good on you, you're nearly ready for the buying stage. To decide what you need, you again have to review what you have. This is the time to rid your closet of all those items that didn't fit (and don't delude yourself that you'll lose the ten pounds required to get into that dress again), or that didn't look good on you. Give all of these items away: to friends, to a local charity, or sell them at a garage sale.

Everything that isn't immediately wearable should be distributed into one of the three categories above. If there are items of clothing you wish to keep for sentimental value, such as your first prom dress or your wedding dress, do so, but these items should comprise the smallest part of your closet space. It's a better idea to pack them carefully for storage in an area other than that used for your everyday wardrobe, such as a basement, attic, or guest room closet.

Include in the pile of clothing to be discarded those items you've not worn for at least a year, no matter how good they still are. If you've not worn a particular outfit for some time that's a pretty good indication that there is something wrong with it for you. It may be an unflattering color or fit poorly. You may always have felt uncomfortable in it, for perhaps undefinable reasons, and so left it hanging in the closet. It's not very likely that you'll wear it again in the near future, so discard it now.

If you take your discarded clothing to a social service agency, be certain to get a receipt for the donation with the estimated value of the clothes clearly stated. That way you can deduct the amount as a charitable contribution from your taxes.

Using the idea proposed by many experts on women's clothing, the object is to develop a "capsule wardrobe." The capsule wardrobe idea is that you will have from 40–60 different outfits with a basic wardrobe consisting of:

- 2 jackets
- 3 skirts
- 4 blouses
- 2 sweaters
- 1 dress

That's barely one side of a walk-in closet, and most of us have many more clothes than that. With those items in your closet, you have a basic, go everywhere, do everything kind of wardrobe. Selecting the right components for your wardrobe will demonstrate your fashion sense, if those 12 pieces, in whatever combination, are items that always look best on you.

Your current wardrobe already may contain the 12 basic pieces. Trying on various combinations of the clothes you already have will help you decide what else you may need to buy to tie things together. You may only need to buy a blouse that will dress up your basic blue suit. Keep accessories in mind as you try out all the various combinations in your wardrobe—will a belt in fashionable metallic spruce up your dress, or skirt and blouse combo?

With your basic wardrobe in place, accessories can be used to dress up or dress down your look, and to add variety to your daily dressing. Accessories often aren't as costly as larger clothing times, so you may want to splurge on an accessory item that is faddish.

Buying Clothes

Now that you know what you need to complete your entire working wardrobe, you're ready to go shopping. Take a list with you. The list should describe specifically each item you're looking for: what color, style, length, and so on. What you buy must coordinate with what you already have. A list will help you identify in detail the items you need to add to your existing wardrobe.

Take the time to look for exactly the right thing. You know by now what looks good on you, so you can wait until you find it. No more settling for second best, only to find that second best really doesn't serve the purpose at all.

In *The Woman's Dress for Success Book*, well-known clothing consultant for industry John T. Molloy offers several tips for buying clothes.[9] Molloy suggests that the woman buying clothes:

- compare the price with anticipated use
- buy on sale
- be certain that markdowns are legitimate
- buy clothes with a local merchant's label not clothes with designer labels
- include cost of upkeep in the cost of clothes
- buy at discount stores or factory outlets.

Comparing the price of an item with its anticipated use will keep you from spending too much money on impractical items. Items for everyday wear, whether for work or home, can and should cost more than items for occasional evenings out.

Buying items at the end of the season will save you money. Other excellent times for clothing sales can be determined by carefully watching newspaper ads.

Making sure that markdowns are legitimate involves organizing your shopping habits. Write down items of clothing in which you are interested.

Be certain you note the manufacturer, the size, color, style, and price. Then, when you see the item on sale you can compare the original price with the sale price. This is particularly valuable if you're shopping in a "discount" clothing store: if you're prepared with facts and figures, you will then know whether an item really is "half-price." Take along a pocket calculator when you shop at sales that advertise percentage markdowns (25 percent, 30 percent, one-third off). Occasionally, the markdowns are not correctly calculated by the store personnel, and you'll want to be certain you're not overcharged for a sale item.

Molloy suggests that clothing or department store buyers are careful about what items of clothing display the store brand.[10] Knowing this will tell you that items with a local merchant's label are more likely to be high quality than those from other merchants.

Prices for clothes with designer labels generally are higher. If you want to buy designer label clothes, look for an outlet store that carries the brand name you want and be certain the prices really are marked down from those in department or other clothing stores before you buy.

If an item of clothing must be dry cleaned, the upkeep of the garment will add to the cost of the garment. If an item has to be washed by hand, the cost of the garment is increased by the amount of your time necessary for its upkeep.

Shopping at outlet stores can decrease the cost of buying clothes. In many of these stores, clothing is reduced by one-half. In some, many of the items offered for sale are "seconds" or "irregulars." Be certain you carefully inspect such garments. You will have to live with whatever it is that makes the garment a second or an irregular, and it's no bargain if you buy something on sale and never wear it because it's defective. It's generally a good idea to shop often at discount stores so you get to know the merchandise and you are there shortly after the really good bargains arrive.

Besides your basic wardrobe for your professional life, you will need clothes for your personal life, such as casual pants and tops and evening wear. You also may need clothes for different seasons, but the principles for your wardrobe of clothes for whatever season are the same.

Once you make this initial effort to plan and organize your wardrobe, you'll find that clothes buying takes much less time and money. You won't be buying styles that will be outdated in a short time, except perhaps for accessories. Since you will be primarily buying good quality clothes, you'll find you won't have to replace them as frequently as poorer quality items.

If your job requires travel, you will be pleased to learn how efficiently your wardrobe can be packed. You also will have the advantage of being well dressed for all occasions while away from home, with a minimum of preparation.

Hairstyle

Your hairstyle is an important part of how you look. It should be flattering. A good hairstyle will be easy to care for and will work for all occasions. It's probably best not to be a slave to the fashionable hairstyles, but to select a style that is best for your face and your life style.

One way to do this is to make an appointment with a well-known hairdresser. If there isn't one in your city or town you may want to wait until you're on vacation or at a convention in a large city when you can get into a well-known hairstylist's salon. Make the appointment with the well-known person, not his or her assistants; for the price you will pay, you will want the person himself or herself.

Ask for a hairstyle that will compliment you. Don't take in a picture from a magazine and ask to be made over to resemble the person in the picture. The hairstylist should work with you to determine the most appropriate style for you.

If you like the style you leave with, have someone take pictures of your hair from all angles. Armed with these pictures you can go to a local beauty salon for future haircuts without having the expense of the well-known hairstylist.

If you decide to select your own hairstyle and have it done at your local beauty salon, scan the magazines for hairstyles you like. Take into consideration the person's hair type in the pictures you like in comparison with your own. If you don't have similar hair, the style won't look the same on you. If you find several styles you like, take the pictures to a wig shop and ask to try on wigs with similar hairstyles. That way you can see how a style looks on you before you invest in it permanently. Take a friend with you for feedback on your new look.

Makeup

Makeup also is a significant part of how you look. It is important that your makeup be applied appropriately for the activities you are involved in; for example, daytime and nightime makeup differ.

Younger women generally can get by with wearing lipstick and little else. Women over 45 may feel better with foundation and a touch of rouge in addition to lipstick.

Makeup should not be obvious. For that reason, eye shadow and eye liner should be reserved for evening wear. Lipstick colors should be muted.

Again, your colleagues are a good source of feedback about your makeup. There also are people at beauty salons and cosmetic counters in department stores who will assist you in selecting makeup to fit your complexion.

If you choose to have your hairstyle done by a well-known hairdresser, ask if makeup consultation is available. In that way, you can benefit from both services at the same time.

Though the makeup consultants will do your face in a flattering manner, you may feel that the amount of makeup used is excessive. You can still initially benefit from their expertise, however, and once you're applying the makeup on your own, modify the amount of makeup you use thereafter.

GETTING STARTED

As mentioned, the first step in beginning to network is realizing that you need help in getting what you want in your professional life. This involves thinking and acting in ways that most of us did not learn as we were growing up as girls. It involves responding to people and situations in a proactive rather than reactive manner. Simply stated, it means taking the initiative in influencing events that shape our professional lives rather than merely allowing things to happen to us.

Many of us believe that things that occur in our work environment cannot be controlled by our actions. We feel that most of the situations that happen are beyond the scope of our influence; they are impersonal happenings that have an impact on us but, in contrast, on which we could not possibly have had an impact.

Individuals knowledgeable about systems and the way they work would effectively refute that kind of thinking. In many instances, the right action taken at the right time can forestall an event or dilute its effects, particularly if those effects are perceived by us as negative ones.

Much of the problem with thinking that events are controlled by factors external to us is a result of not being aware of what goes on in our work setting. Nurses are very knowledgeable about their particular job responsibilities. They are very competent in the provision of direct nursing care, in teaching in a school of nursing, in administering a health care facility, but their knowledge and competence in relation to the employing environment ends there. Many nurses are not aware of how decisions are made in their employing agency, nor are they aware of how they could work to affect those decisions being made, particularly those that directly affect them.

The second step, then, in becoming skillful at networking is to become aware of what is going on around you in your professional employment setting. Find out who has the power where you work. Who is responsible for making decisions and whose decisions, when made, stick? Whose decisions can, and often do, get remanded? Who has input into the decision-making process? Who is part of the informal power in the organization (not necessarily depicted as the formal authority on the table of organization). Chances are, you already know much of this information; you've just not had occasion to think about it in terms of a framework for your efforts at networking.

IDENTIFYING YOUR EXISTING NETWORKS

As you sharpen your awareness skills on the job you'll begin to note who is in your existing networks. Don't limit yourself just to individuals with whom you currently work. Consider all individuals with whom you have had or do have contact. Consider your friends, on and off the job, classmates from your basic nursing education program and others such as from high school, college, continuing education courses, or academic classes that you may have taken but were not part of a formal degree program.

Consider individuals in your spouse's or family's circle of friends. Count also individuals whom you know from church or your children's school activities. Your list should be extensive; write down as many names as you can think of. You'll pare the list of your contacts down later, but for now you need to note as many individuals as possible.

When you consider your "professional" or "at work" network, start by asking yourself these questions: With whom do you spend most of your time? Whom do you consult for advice on problems? In whom do you confide successes? To whom do you go when you want something done? Include all of these individuals as part of your existing networks.

Next, define your existing networks in three spheres:

- your vertical, upward network
- your horizontal network
- your vertical, downward network

A vertical, upward network consists of those individuals who are above you in terms of status or position.

The horizontal network is comprised of your peers or colleagues with whom you work or participate in other professional activities, such as membership in a state nurses' association or community service.

Your vertical, downward network is composed of those individuals who are below you in terms of status or position. Generally, these are individuals to whom you provide support, assistance, and counsel.

Recognizing and then defining your existing network is one element in getting started. You then will need to determine how effective your existing networks are. Many of the individuals you identified as contacts you haven't kept in touch with over time, for example, those persons with whom you went to high school or through your nursing program. At a later step in the process you'll have to decide about reinstituting contact but for now focus on those individuals with whom you maintain contact, however infrequent.

When assessing the effectiveness of your network of contacts, you will have to ask some hard questions of yourself. Do you use the contacts who are a part of your network to result in your professional gain? Or do you use your time with them, particularly those contacts with whom you work, for gossip, to tell tales, to pass the time of day, or a myriad of other such interactions that won't serve your purposes very effectively? Normal social conversation has a place in the process of networking, but idle conversation with no apparent purpose for either participant does not. Valuable time and energy are wasted on such communication of little ultimate value.

In reviewing your professional networks, particularly your "at work" network, you may note that you already have the organization's "movers and shakers," those people who can help you get what you want, in your network. If not, you can learn networking strategies that will help you include those people in your expanded networks.

EXPANDING YOUR NETWORKS

Next, you'll have to identify the networks you'll need in order to get where you want to be professionally. Networking is the process of making and using contacts, but it doesn't involve indiscriminately adding people to your networks. The contacts you make should have a focus. You should have a purpose in mind for expanding a network to obtain additional contacts. At this point, you may not have a clear idea of exactly who the persons are who may be of most assistance to you, but you probably can identify those individuals by position.

For example, if you want to advance to a supervisory position in a hospital, those nurses already in administrative positions in that institution most likely can be of most assistance to you. If you want to publish, it would be helpful to know an editor or publisher. If you want to teach in continuing education programs, you would want to meet those individuals who are administrators or directors of continuing education programs in colleges or universities.

Once you've decided who should be in your network, you must decide how to make contact with them. There are four ways to make contact:

- Make a phone call
- Write a letter
- Arrange a face-to-face meeting
- Get a referral

You probably will select the means for meeting a contact based on your comfort level. It may be easiest to pick up the phone and call the individual. You might say "Hello, this is Martha Maxwell. I'm calling because I'm interested in doing my master's thesis on baccalaureate nurses' perceptions of role responsibilities in comparison with perceptions of associate degree nurses. I read several of the articles you've published on the subject. Would you be able to spend some time discussing my thesis topic with me?"

You may be more comfortable with writing a letter to the person whom you wish to meet. The letter should contain some brief information about who you are and why you are contacting the individual. You may send a copy of your curriculum vitae along with the letter if appropriate. For example, if you are directing the letter to the head of the continuing education program at the local university, and you wish to be asked to teach educational offerings, a copy of your vitae will illustrate your educational and experiential qualifications for teaching, as well as indicate where you've previously taught in continuing education programs.

You may be most comfortable with arranging a face-to-face meeting with a potential contact for your expanded network. Obviously, to do this you must know where those individuals are likely to be. An editor or publisher would be likely to be an exhibitor at a national nursing convention. A continuing education director probably would attend meetings of organizations whose membership is comprised of individuals in similar positions, or he or she might be present at a continuing education offering sponsored by his or her program to introduce the speakers, and so on.

If you're not certain where the people you want to meet might be, then ask around. Individuals in your existing networks can be an excellent source of that information. Read newspapers, journals, and other publications to see where nationally known people are appearing as speakers.

Find out what charities and other activities the people you want to meet are involved in. Volunteer your services for the same charity. You may be assigned to work on the same committee as the person you've identified as potentially being most helpful to you.

Attend meetings of the groups where individuals you want to add to your expanded networks also may be. Putting yourself in situations where the people are whom you want to meet is a good way to make contacts.

Another excellent way to meet those individuals whom you wish to meet is to be referred to them by someone else. Here your existing network can be of use. Ask around. Does anyone in your network know an editor? Would he or she be willing to let you use his or her name when you meet the editor? In this case, you can approach the individual with a bit more assurance that you will be well received.

For example, a nurse says to an editor at a book exhibit at a national nurses' meeting: "Mrs. James, at the suggestion of Diane Murray, I would like to talk with you about an idea I have for writing a book. When would it be convenient for you to meet with me during this conference?"

In order to meet contacts, you may wish to use a combination of the four approaches identified. You may phone first, then follow up by arranging a face-to-face meeting. In that instance, you can begin the conversation with your potential contact by saying something like "Good afternoon. I'm Martha Maxwell; we spoke recently on the telephone when I called to discuss my master's thesis. It's good to see you. Will you perhaps have some free time during the convention to talk with me?"

GETTING ORGANIZED

Networking is a systematized way of meeting and using contacts to help you advance professionally. It works best when treated as a precise science, rather than haphazardly. As you meet individuals you wish to add to your network, keep a record of their names and other vital information.

One excellent way of keeping networking records is through the exchange of business cards. When you meet people, ask for a business card. Have your own business cards to exchange. If you have not had business cards before, make a visit to a local print shop where they can be made to order.

Select a good quality paper. Most business cards are white but an off-white or cream color is just as suitable. Avoid vividly colored paper. Black or dark blue ink is preferable to more trendy colors. Your business card should contain, at a minimum, your

- name
- credentials
- place of business
- business address
- business phone

Your name should be centered on the card. Avoid using titles such as Mrs. or Dr. before your name.

You may wish to include your title, but do so only if your title is unlikely to change. If your title is likely to change, leave it off, as it's costly to purchase cards frequently.

If you prefer being contacted at home rather than at your business address or phone, include your home address and telephone number. You may want to use your home address and phone number if you are planning to change employment settings in the near future or any time before your supply of cards is exhausted.

If any of the information on your business card should change, purchase more cards. Don't strike through outdated information and write in the correct information with pen or pencil. The cost of buying a new supply of cards is far less than the cost of making a poor impression!

When you receive a business card, you may wish to make notes to yourself on the reverse side of the card. These notes can include (1) where you met the person, (2) the content of your conversation, and (3) any follow-up necessary.

Keep the business cards you collect in an organized fashion for easy reference. You may wish to purchase a notebook (at office supply or stationery stores) designed for the purpose of storing business cards. You may find an ordinary file box suitable for your storage needs.

Organizing the cards by topic probably will be the most productive for your networking efforts. For example, a continuing educator's business card collection may be organized under such topic headings as:

- potential clinical faculty (although this heading may have to be further subdivided by area of clinical expertise)
- evaluation
- grantsmanship
- marketing

A nursing service administrator's topic headings may look more like:

- JCAH requirements
- staffing
- budgeting
- cost containment
- computers
- nursing process

Your system may be similar to these or completely different. Whatever system you use, it needs only to be organized so that you can avail yourself of the contacts you've made when you need to.

If you find that the contacts you need to make are people in another already-existing network of which you are not a member, then become part of that network. You may wish to start your own network in order to involve those people who can be of most use to you and to one another.

One point must be made here. As Welch notes in *Networking*, you don't necessarily need to like the people with whom you network.[11] A network may be composed of your friends, but the network doesn't need to be reserved exclusively for friends. Those people you would refer to as "colleagues," "acquaintances," and others can be part of your network. This seems to be less problematic for men; they can easily conduct business with individuals who are not their friends; women, however, seem to mix their personal feelings in with their professional lives more often.

You may find that, because of your mutual interests, you do make friends with many of the individuals with whom you network. This is certainly a bonus for you. The important consideration is that you do not expect that friendship will be necessary for you to be successful in your networking efforts.

INITIAL NETWORKING ATTEMPTS

A common place for networking is at a meeting, such as a business or trade convention, where the individuals with whom you wish to network are present. Wear your name tag at all times, so people won't have to guess or ask who you are. Not wearing your name tag may cause some individuals, knowing that you look familiar and wondering where they've met you, to be interested enough to approach you. But such ploys also can have the opposite effect. In order not to be embarrassed because they ought to know you and they can't remember you, they avoid you.

When you walk up to someone to introduce yourself, even though you are wearing a name tag, say your name. Hearing your name aloud eliminates any uncertainty about the correct pronunciation and reinforces the individual's remembering you.

Be sure you pronounce your name clearly and loudly enough for the individual to hear you correctly. Because we are so familiar with our own names and the way they sound, we often mumble or introduce ourselves inarticulately. It can be helpful to practice introducing yourself in a mirror, so that you are aware of how you appear to others.

If you know the individual but haven't seen him or her for some time, it's a good idea to give your name along with some hint about where you met, particularly if there's a possibility that the individual may not remember you: "Hello, Mary, I haven't seen you since the nursing manpower meeting in Chicago in July last year. How have you been?" or "Dr. Sample, I'm Angela Throop; we met last year after your presentation in San Francisco. We talked briefly about your theories on nurse retention. In the meantime I've done some study on my own. I'd like to tell you some of the reasons I found that influenced nurse retention. Would you be free to have a drink and talk now?"

The individuals in these illustrations were networking effectively. They were making contacts and communicating with others about matters of interest and importance to them. As you start your networking efforts toward meeting your own goals, you will recognize the need for effective communication skills.

COMMUNICATION SKILLS

A person's life, both personally and professionally, depends upon the ability to make thoughts, feelings, and needs known to others. The individual also has to be receptive to others as they make known their thoughts, feelings, and needs.

Communication is the result of individuals' attempts to share their thoughts, feelings, and needs with each other. In the simplest terms, communication is the sending and receiving of messages. Both elements (sending and receiving) must be present for communication to occur, although not all transmission and reception of messages is communication. Occasionally, the message is not clearly sent or is distorted as it is received. In that case, communication has not occurred.

In order to network effectively, you need to be able to transmit messages as you mean them. You also must be able to receive messages from others as they intend them. In short, you must be able to communicate well.

Good communication skills require that the individual possess several interpersonal characteristics.[12] These are:

- a strong self-concept
- ability to listen
- clear expression
- ability to cope with anger
- ability to disclose self

All of these characteristics are present to some extent in each individual. It is important to assess which of these you currently possess and which you need to improve upon, so that your communication can be as effective as possible.

Self-Concept

An individual's self-concept is formed early in life. Individuals begin to perceive themselves based on how others perceive them. If they are loved, they perceive themselves as lovable; if they are accepted, they perceive themselves as acceptable.

Individuals see their world through their concept of themselves. The self-concept acts as a filter through which communication is sent and received. If an individual has a strong self-concept, his or her communication will be direct, secure, and satisfying. On the other hand, if an individual's self-concept is weak, his or her communication will be insecure and timid. That individual will have trouble voicing opinions, accepting criticism, and expressing feelings.

Listening

The ability to listen is an essential component of effective communication. Listening is an active skill, which requires effort on the part of the listener to obtain the real meaning of what the speaker is saying. Listening is a skill that can be acquired (or improved upon) through practice. Techniques to practice that can improve an individual's ability to listen include:

- having a reason or purpose for listening
- eliminating distractions that interfere with listening (such as having the television or radio on in the background)
- trying to elicit the important content of what the speaker is saying
- recognizing that the rate of speech is 100–150 words per minute and the rate of thought is 400–500 words per minute, so that the listener resists thinking of a response while the speaker is speaking
- rephrasing what the speaker has said before answering

The effective listener interacts with the speaker in a meaningful fashion so that the conversation includes both of them at the same time, instead of being parallel conversations. Effective listening occurs when the listener clearly understands the speaker's message.

Clarity of Expression

The ability to express oneself clearly is another component of effective communication skills. Many people assume that others understand the meaning behind what they are saying without ever checking it out. Much everyday speech is careless and unclear. Precision in speech patterns is necessary for others to understand what we mean.

Poor communicators assume that others understand what they say. They operate on the assumption that what they said was understood in the way they meant it to be. Those listening, in turn, operate on what it was they thought the speaker was saying. The result is complete misunderstanding.

The person who communicates well has a clear idea of what he or she is trying to say. After saying it, he or she uses feedback techniques to ensure that the listener has a clear idea of what was said. If the feedback indicates that the message was not clear, the speaker can elaborate or clarify as necessary to communicate the message as intended.

Coping with Anger

Anger is a difficult emotion for many to express. Inability to cope with angry feelings often leads to breakdowns in communication. Some people cope with their anger by suppressing it, which may result in a physical response such as ulcers. Others explode at the slightest provocation. Still others avoid disagreements at all costs; they become upset at the slightest indication that there may be conflict.

None of these people is able to cope with angry feelings in a constructive fashion. Those angry feelings must be communicated in order to establish or maintain good relationships with others. Some guidelines that may be helpful in the expression of feelings, including angry ones are:

- know what your emotions are
- admit having your emotions
- accept responsibility for your emotions
- find out what your emotions mean
- tell others about your emotions
- integrate your emotions as part of your self
- learn from your emotions so that you may grow

Self-Disclosure

Self-disclosure is necessary for effective communication. Communication experts say that individuals cannot really communicate with each other unless they engage in self-disclosure. Self-disclosure is a mutual process—the more individuals know about each other, the more effectively they are able to communicate with each other. A person's ability to disclose himself or herself to others is a sign of a healthy personality, a reflection of an individual with a strong self-concept.

Many people are concerned about disclosing themselves to others for fear of rejection. This feeling of fear prevents them from developing a trusting relationship with others. An effective communicator is one who can establish an atmosphere of trust in which others can feel comfortable in disclosing themselves.

The ultimate goal of effective communication will be reached if an individual possesses the necessary interpersonal characteristics. Those that the individual does not now have can be learned in order to have the good communication skills necessary to network effectively.

COMMUNICATION IN NETWORKING

Once you have good communication skills, you will need to be aware of those particular communication skills that are part of the networking process. These are (1) becoming aware of networking talk and (2) learning what not to talk about when networking.

Networking talk is primarily professional talk. Networking conversations focus mainly on employment-related topics. Casual, warm-up remarks typically are about current events, food, movies, books, and other leisure-time activities.

Good warm-up topics include comments on what you are experiencing together at the present. Such opening remarks can be about the meeting you are both attending: "Wasn't that a great keynote address? I thought it particularly meaningful when she described continuing education as being on the cutting edge of the profession. That description takes us beyond merely planning programs for nurses, doesn't it?" The other individual then can respond to your opening statement and the conversation ensues.

In order to be able to converse knowledgeably about current events, you may have to read the local newspapers or magazines. If there are topics that you know are of particular interest to the persons you wish to meet, prepare yourself with information about those topics. Avoid learning about such topics just to impress those persons; better to profess ignorance and have the person teach you than to be thought to be "showing off" or get in over your head by not being able to maintain your end of the conversation. The key to being a good conversationalist is to be able to discuss issues other than those pertaining only to your own field.

Learning what not to talk about is as important as learning how to talk networking talk. One used to hear that discussions about religion and politics were taboo. In networking, families and children generally are not topics of conversation between contacts. Gossip and idle stories about others definitely are not appropriate networking talk.

Avoid making negative or critical comments about other people. When you continuously downgrade others, your listeners may wonder what you say about them when they're not with you. It's not helpful to get a reputation for being a criticizer. A friend once suggested a useful technique when you find yourself saying too many negative things about a person: say three positive things about the person before you allow yourself to say one negative thing. Using that technique in your current everyday conversations will help you become aware of how negative you are about others. Being aware of your behavior is the necessary first step in being able to subsequently change it.

If it is important that you do convey negative information about another person in the course of your networking, try to do it as objectively as possible. Phrase your comments in as constructive a manner as you can. Avoid overkill—you need not emphasize your point with innumerable examples for your listener to get the gist of your criticism.

Avoid being overly critical of your work and, more particularly, your boss. Your listener may wonder if it's such a terrible place in which to work why are you still working there? In essence, your criticism may say more about you than it says about what you are criticizing.

SUMMARY

Networking is easy to do. It takes some time to get organized and begin to network effectively. The time devoted to describing your existing networks is well spent, however, as it ultimately allows you to see who you need to add to your networks in order to get what you want.

Getting what you want involves being prepared to network skillfully. In order to do that, you must have the "tools of the trade." You have to have a vitae or resume to let people know who you are and why they want you for a particular professional opportunity.

You have to dress well so that you look appropriate for the role you are to be filling. Stylish clothing helps you give the appearance of a successful, competent woman.

Finally, you have to be willing to try networking to see how well it works for you. You must be willing to risk being a bit nervous as you attempt to network the first few times. There may be some initial failures as you try your skills. The ultimate benefits you discover as a result of your networking activities, however, will convince you that all of the

women who are members of networks really have found the key to professional success. And, once you begin networking, you will have found it
for yourself!

NOTES

1. Ronald L. Krannich and William J. Banis, *High Impact Resumes & Letters* (Chesapeake, Va.: Progressive Concepts, 1982), p. 11.

2. Ibid., p. 12.

3. Ibid., p. 10.

4. B. Joan Newcomb and Patricia A. Murphy, "The Curriculum Vitae—What It Is and What It Is Not," *Nursing Outlook* 27, no. 9 (September 1979): 580–583.

5. Krannich and Banis, *High Impact Resumes & Letters*, p. 21.

6. Ibid., p. 21.

7. Ibid., pp. 43–63.

8. Richard Germann and Peter Arnold, *Bernard Haldane Associates' Job & Career Building* (New York: Harper & Row, 1980), pp. 54–55.

9. John T. Molloy, *The Woman's Dress For Success Book* (New York: Warner Books, 1977), pp. 167–171.

10. *Ibid.* p. 168.

11. Mary Scott Welch, *Networking* (New York: Harcourt Brace Jovanovich, 1980), p. 76.

12. Myron R. Chartier, "Five Components Contributing to Effective Interpersonal Communications," *The 1974 Annual Handbook for Group Facilitators* (La Jolla, Calif.: University Associates), pp. 125–128.

Chapter 3

Starting a Network

Once you have decided that networking is for you, you may realize that your already-existing networks won't accomplish what you want. You also may realize that expanding your networks by a few, or many, members still won't be helpful in attaining your goals. In that case, you may have to start a network of your own.

It's not difficult to start a network; it just takes time and energy. Women in all positions and in all fields of work have started their own networks. They, too, felt that their existing opportunities for networking did not meet their needs. So, they started a network that would provide them with exactly what they needed. You can, too!

There are several steps to follow in the process of starting a new network. These steps include:

- establishing the need
- determining the membership
- setting the meeting
- conducting the meeting
- determining the network's directions
- following up on necessary actions
- formalizing the network

ESTABLISHING THE NEED FOR A NETWORK

You may have identified the need for a network to achieve a certain professional goal of yours. It may well be that others share the same need and would be interested in a network that would be of assistance in the attainment of that specific goal.

In order to establish a new network, you must have an apparent need for the group. Start with a few of your friends or colleagues, particularly those who you think may share your professional goals. Talk with them individually or in a small group about the new network you think is necessary. In the process of setting up the network at Equitable, Alina Novak reported talking with quite a few other female employees in a "series of one-to-one lunches" to discuss their interest in the kind of group she thought was needed at Equitable.[1]

Even if you're not in a position to arrange for such luncheon meetings with the persons you think may be interested in your new network, you can accomplish the same thing by talking with your nursing colleagues at work, or at times other than work when you are together. The important thing is to establish others' need for the new network as well as your own.

Discuss your ideas for a new network with as many individuals as possible. The purpose of these discussions is to elicit interest in a new network and to develop a core group of persons who will help you form the network. During these discussions, be as open and accepting of new ideas and perceptions as you can. Although the network is your idea, it may be that some of the ideas of your friends improve your thinking tremendously.

DETERMINING THE MEMBERSHIP

Once you have identified a core group of three or four individuals who will help you initiate the new network, you need to decide who else will be members of the new group. Each of you should develop a list of people who should be invited to join the network. If you can't identify these individuals by name, then indicate who should be invited by position, for example, a hospital administrator, an attorney, an accountant, and so on. Each of you should identify as many potential members as possible.

Try to develop your membership lists separately at first, and then meet together to merge your lists. Hearing the names or positions of those all of you have identified may generate some additional names or positions. These lists of members should be as comprehensive as possible.

In her book *Networking,* Mary Scott Welch suggests that among the potential members of a new network, you include "stars" and "known doers."[2] Stars are defined as those individuals who are well known and successful in their fields. These people will help attract members to your new network. Welch suggests that the stars be made members of the network's advisory committee if they are not willing to become members of the network itself.

Doers are defined as those individuals who get things done. They are the workers in an organization who seem to accomplish more than anyone else. Welch suggests that these individuals be involved to assist in getting the network established.

Your core group of individuals can accomplish the same purpose as involving known doers. Particularly if the core group is enthusiastic about the prospect of a new network, they will be energetic in getting it started.

Now you've established an idea of who will be initially asked to join the new network. You may continue to add members to the network as you go along, but the initial membership roster is set. At least for the first meeting, those who are to attend have been identified. It's time to set the meeting date and time.

SETTING THE INITIAL MEETING

You and your core group now must establish the first meeting date, time, and location. Try to avoid as many conflicting occasions as possible, knowing, of course, that you won't be able to avoid everything that's going on that may conflict with your meeting. Recognize, too, that the individuals you will invite to your meeting are adults who may have other priorities for that day and time than attending your meeting.

Knowing that you will never be able to ensure a meeting date that accommodates everyone, set the date for at least the first meeting. Those individuals in attendance at that meeting can set subsequent meeting dates for themselves.

Try to select a meeting time that will be most convenient for everyone. Again, meeting times may have to be changed later by the members of the network. Allow sufficient time to accomplish the business of beginning the new network. At least two hours is the minimum to be allotted for the first meeting.

The meeting location has to be determined at this time also. If you wish to include a social element along with the business of establishing a new network, one of the core group members may have the meeting at his or her home. If the anticipated attendance is too large for a meeting at someone's home, you may have to find another place to meet.

There are a number of places where groups can meet free of charge. Churches, public libraries, and auditoriums in shopping center malls are examples. The site chosen should be large enough for the group to meet comfortably.

The place chosen should be "neutral" for the group members. For example, nurses who are meeting to establish a network for collective bargaining purposes might not want to meet at their hospital or other place of employment. Some nurses might not want to meet at the local university, and some may not wish to use a church basement. Be sensitive to the wishes of the group. Your core group can assist you with the selection of the meeting place.

The meeting place should be centrally located for ease of access. If the meeting is at night, lighted parking close to the building is necessary. Parking should be as convenient to the meeting location as possible. If possible, choose a location where there is security.

If all those individuals attending the meeting are not familiar with the meeting location, prepare a map or a written set of directions to send with the meeting invitations. The map or directions should be easy to follow.

Next, draw up a meeting agenda. The agenda should list all of the topics for discussion at the meeting. It is a good idea to put the items for discussion on the agenda in order of priority, so that the meeting doesn't end with the most important items yet to be discussed. This will also help to eliminate the possibility that some people may leave the meeting a bit early and all the important items are handled after they leave.

You may wish to indicate a specific amount of time on the agenda for discussion of each of the topics so that there is some direction for the group and all the items to be discussed are addressed in the meeting as planned. You may wish to omit the time allocation, however, if you feel the group would be constrained by those limits.

Send all of the materials (meeting invitation, agenda, and map) to those individuals you and the core group identified as potential members of the new network. The materials should be sent as far in advance of the meeting as possible so that people can clear their calendars to attend.

The materials should be neatly typed and duplicated. If there is not secretarial assistance available, you may wish to neatly handwrite the letter of invitation and agenda. Copies can be obtained inexpensively from a photocopy shop. The cost of mailing invitations can be reduced somewhat if the core group members distribute some invitations by hand.

Members of the core group may have to finance the cost of printing and postage for the initial meeting. You may plan to ask at the first meeting for contributions from those in attendance to help in defraying the costs of the initial meeting.

Once the meeting date, time, and location have been set, your next step is to prepare to conduct the meeting. Careful preparation may well spell the difference between success and failure in relation to the establishment of the new network.

CONDUCTING THE MEETING

In preparing to conduct the first meeting of the new network, you will need to select a chairperson or leader for the group. It may be that you are the most appropriate individual to assume that role, particularly since the new network was your idea. If you are uncertain about your ability to serve as chairperson for the first meeting, and you think that another member of the core group would be better suited for that role, it might be best for you to defer the leadership role to the other individual.

Before the meeting, check the room setup. You probably will want the tables and chairs to be arranged informally. Choose "rounds" if possible, so that a group of six to eight individuals is seated around one table. "Classroom" style, where individuals are seated in rows, often contributes to a formal meeting format, where there are questions and answers rather than open and free participation in discussion.

For at least the first meeting, have individuals "register." If it is not possible for one of the members of the core group to register individuals as they arrive at the meeting, then a place should be set aside for self-registration. A notebook can be set out on a table for each person to sign his or her name, address, and phone number. Include instructions so that each indicates his or her preferred mailing address for future network communications.

You and the other members of your core group should greet each of the persons arriving. Circulate around the room before the meeting starts so that you identify yourselves to those present and make them feel welcome.

Have refreshments available if at all possible. You can provide hot water in a coffee pot along with instant coffee and tea bags. Lemonade or soft drinks are nice during afternoon meetings in the warmer months. If you are able to provide them, there can be cookies or other snacks available.

Start the meeting with introductions. Introduce yourself to the group members and ask that they introduce themselves to you and to one another. If most of the individuals present do not know one another, you may wish to use a "get-acquainted" exercise. Such an exercise is useful in helping those present get to know one another more rapidly than they would if left to their own devices. If some of the decisions to be made at the first meeting require that the group be fairly cohesive, the get-acquainted exercise will be a necessary tool.

One such get-acquainted exercise is described as the "cocktail party mix" by Pfeiffer and Jones.[3] In this exercise, participants are given a sheet of paper or an index card on which they write three to five key characteristics that describe them. These characteristics can be personality traits, hobbies, or current interests they are pursuing. The key dimensions of their personalities are written on the paper or card in a legible manner so that others can easily read them.

The paper or card then is pinned to the individuals, who circulate around the room in cocktail party fashion. A specific time is allotted for everyone present to read what others have written about themselves without speaking.

After this silent period of circulation, the participants are encouraged to return to the two or three individuals whose key characteristics interested them. At this stage, then, the participants circulate again, stopping to chat when they see an individual whose card interests them. An effort should be made to allow enough time for each person to talk with at least three or four others in the room.

Variations on this cocktail party mix also can be used. In one variation, participants are given a 9-inch paper plate instead of a sheet of paper or index card. They then are told that the paper plate represents a "pie" of their time. They are requested to describe how they spend their time by drawing "slices" on the pie. In one instance, the largest slice comprises work, the next largest care of the home, such as cooking and cleaning, then hobbies, such as folk dancing, and so on. The participants then circulate in the room comparing and contrasting their own with others' pies, again frequently stopping to chat.

Using a human relations exercise, such as the cocktail party mix, will facilitate those present getting to know one another. When the meeting is called to order, often participants will sit with people with whom they talked during the exercise. Thus, friendships and alliances begin to be formed in the new network.

Name tags also are helpful in the getting-acquainted process. Also useful are large index cards (5 × 9) folded in half, on which participants print their names with a felt tip pen. When these cards are placed in front of all the persons at the table, it is easier to identify them and easier for the chairperson or group leader to remember names.

It probably will be helpful to have extra copies of the agenda handy as you start the meeting. Someone may have forgotten his or hers and there could be "drop-ins," individuals who heard about the new network and were interested enough to come to the meeting.

Begin the meeting by explaining how you decided to form the network. Tell those present specifically what you thought was needed and how you thought those needs could be met through the formation of the new network. Identify clearly the process you followed to initiate this meeting. Tell those present how the core group was formed.

Each of the participants will be curious about how he or she was chosen to become part of the network. Describe how they were selected to be invited to the meeting. You may have to repeat this information so that everyone clearly understands. Be prepared to answer questions about why other individuals were not asked to attend the meeting.

You will want to select one individual to take notes of the meetings so that important issues and decisions will be recorded. One of the members of the core group can be the recorder. If you decide to have minutes of the meeting to distribute, the recording may be more formalized than if you just wish to keep track of the important occurrences during the meeting.

Ask participants if they wish to have a listing of those persons in attendance. Be certain that everyone agrees that his or her name and other information can be circulated. Some individuals may prefer that their home telephone numbers not be released. You may need to recirculate the registration list so that corrections and deletions may be made.

Repeat at this point the reasons you thought a new network was important and needed. Those present should contribute their thoughts and ideas on the need for the network. You may be able to manage this discussion with the whole group participating, if the group is relatively small. If the group is large, consider a number of small group discussions, where six to ten individuals discuss the need for the network among themselves. Then, each small group gives a report of its discussion to the group as a whole. In this way you can ensure everyone's participation. Also, those individuals who are reluctant to speak up in a large group may be more comfortable contributing their ideas in a smaller group.

DETERMINING DIRECTIONS

In addition to discussing why you and others present think a new network is necessary, you will want to discuss specifically what you think the network will be able to accomplish. Those who are present and interested in the establishment of a new network will be the ones to give the network some focus and direction.

Though the network was your idea, be cautious about wanting to retain "ownership" of the network after you've involved other interested people. Their ideas of what the network should do may differ greatly from what you envisioned. Try to listen to new ideas and directions for your network with an open mind. It may be that the group's idea of an effective network actually is better and more productive than anything you had thought of alone or with members of the core group. Reserve judgment on the value of others' suggestions if they are different from yours. Some of what the group decides may not correspond with what you would have decided, but your purpose here is to start a network from which others, besides yourself, can and will benefit. Constraining the network too tightly to what will benefit you, and perhaps only you, will not contribute to the formation of an effective network.

Among the other issues you will discuss about the network, you will need to address such topics as:

- membership
- rules for operation or bylaws
- officers or leaders

Membership

If the network you form doesn't have the members it needs, it won't be an effective network. All of the members have to be involved in the network's activities in order for it to be viable. While all of the individuals who attend the first meeting generally are interested in the concept of the network, they may not wish to become active members. You may have to recruit other interested individuals in order to fully establish your network.

On the other hand, you may have more interested individuals than are appropriate for the purposes of your network. In that case, you will have to establish some sort of membership screening process. You may choose to have applications for membership reviewed by several members of the network and applicants chosen who most closely meet the established criteria for membership. You may choose to have membership applications reviewed in meetings of the entire network membership, with a majority vote determining if the individual is accepted into membership.

Whatever method you choose for determining the network membership, it is important that the entire group be involved in making the decision about how members of the network will be selected. One compromise solution, in the event that some of those present at the initial network meeting may not meet the established membership criteria, is to establish a category of "Charter Members." Those who were present at the first meeting, then, become members of the network by virtue of their interest and involvement in the organizational meeting. Subsequent to the first meeting, other interested individuals must meet the criteria in order to become members of the network.

You also may decide that your network will be open to anyone who wishes to join. In that case, the problem of membership is simplified.

Rules for Operation

The group will have to decide about having rules for operation or bylaws for the network. While such documents may be viewed by some as hampering the functioning of the organization, they may be necessary to ensure that the network operates as it was designed to.

Rules for operation are less structured than bylaws. The rules should contain information on:

- functions of the network
- membership
- officers
- nominating and election policies and procedures
- committees, their functions and membership
- revision of the rules

It generally is more efficient to have a small group develop rules for operation or bylaws and bring them to the larger group for discussion and action. If the group chooses to have bylaws, a small group can develop the concepts to be embodied in the bylaws. When the network membership approves those concepts, then a parliamentarian can be engaged to actually write the bylaws in the appropriate language.

Officers

An important component of both rules for operation and bylaws is selection of officers. The members of the network may choose not to have formal nominating and election procedures, but there should be some formalized method established for selecting the network's leadership. For the first few meetings, you or other members of the core group may chair the network meetings. After the organizational work of the group is completed, other officers may be chosen.

At a minimum, the network will need a chairperson and secretary. If there are finances to be maintained, you will need a treasurer if either the chairperson or secretary cannot assume this additional responsibility. You also may wish to have a person designated as the vice-chairperson. That individual would assume responsibility for chairing network meetings in the absence of the chairperson.

The position of chairperson can be rotated throughout the membership of the group. This allows everyone the opportunity to serve as the group's leader, but may result in inconsistent leadership and activity levels for the group. If the secretarial responsibilities are rotated throughout the membership, no one is excessively burdened with note taking, but the records of the network meetings may be inconsistent because of different note-taking styles. If formal minutes are to be kept of the network meetings, a permanent secretary probably is best.

Finally, during the initial meeting, you'll want to address such issues as how often to meet, when to meet again, and such specifics as the date and time of the next meeting. Ending the meeting with a summary of actions taken during the meeting reviews for the group exactly what was accomplished. Identifying follow-up actions and who is responsible for them is helpful. Also listing all items for discussion at future meetings will assist the group to focus on their future tasks and responsibilities.

FOLLOWING UP

Once the initial meeting of the network has been conducted, you probably will find that there are many items that must be taken care of. The members of your core group should be available to assist you with the follow-up tasks, if other members of the network weren't assigned.

Hopefully, the group would have identified an individual to be responsible for the minutes of the meeting. If not, you will have to circulate the record of the meeting to those who were present. You also may want to send a copy of the meeting minutes to those who were invited but were unable to attend.

Perhaps an individual or small group will be responsible for the membership of the network. If not, you may have received some direction from the group about others to invite to join the network. You will need to contact those persons to ascertain their interest in joining the network.

If there was not an arrangements person or committee identified, it will be your responsibility to schedule the location of the next meeting. Refreshments must be obtained, and so on.

You will want to prepare for the meeting well in advance, so that the meeting announcement and agenda can be mailed to those who weren't able to attend the first meeting. The person who took notes during the previous meeting should be relied upon to help establish the next meeting's agenda if it wasn't agreed upon by the group at the conclusion of the previous meeting.

If your network members decided to meet as frequently as every week, you may not have enough time to prepare and mail the meeting minutes in advance of the next meeting. In that case, the minutes can be distributed for review at the beginning of each meeting. All that is necessary from one meeting to the next is that the members, particularly those who weren't present, be reminded of the date and time of the next meeting. If the meeting dates and times are standardized, such as every Wednesday at 7 P.M. or the third Thursday of the month at 2:30 P.M., it may not be necessary to send meeting reminders.

If the network is meeting infrequently, try to mail meeting announcements from four to six weeks in advance of the meeting. That time period is ample for most people to schedule a meeting. Less notice can cause difficulty for people with busy schedules.

FORMALIZING THE NETWORK

Once you've had the initial meeting of your network, you will want to ensure that it continues to be active. You may decide to name the network and actively recruit members. Let others know that the network has been established. Tell people about the network's functions and its future directions.

Try to get publicity for the newly established network in the media, particularly if you are interested in recruiting more members. Getting publicity for your network's activities also may be a good way of receiving donations from individuals and corporations to finance your projects. It is helpful to have women in the media as members of your network. They may be more interested in providing publicity for an activity in which they are personally involved.

During the formalization process, the rules by which the network will operate should be established and approved by the membership. Financial stability for the network should be ensured.

FINANCING THE NETWORK

Financing the network's activities may be problematic. There should be money available to cover the cost of printing the minutes of the meetings and mailing them to members. There also must be money to print and mail meeting announcements. Refreshments must be paid for, although members of the network may rotate assignments for bringing the refreshments. Funds can be obtained for the network activities by collecting a small fee from each person attending a meeting when they register. Or, all of the individuals at the meeting can be asked to contribute whatever amount they wish to the network treasury. Both of these ways will provide funds, but may not result in adequate amounts to continue network activities, except on a meeting-to-meeting basis.

Members may wish to consider a dues structure in order to adequately finance the network. If you do decide to charge dues for membership, be certain you check state and local laws governing organizations such as your network.

The dues should be set at the lowest possible level in order not to discourage potential members. Dues money can be maintained in an interest-bearing savings account, with only the funds necessary for immediate use transferred into a checking account. Fund-raising projects can be attempted to earn money for the network's activities.

Again, small groups are most effective in outlining plans for financing the network. The larger group then can take appropriate action on the various plans presented. It is helpful to involve women who work in financial institutions, such as banks or brokerage houses, in the financial aspects of the network.

LONG-RANGE PLANNING

Long-range planning for network activities is an essential component to ensure the continuation of the network. Among the matters involved in long-range planning are:

- membership recruitment and retention
- meeting schedule and content

Membership Matters

If your new network is to work and to continue to exist and prosper, there must continue to be members. The initial members who joined the network may continue to be actively involved throughout the life of the network, but there may be attrition of these members for reasons beyond your control. Members may move away from the area or obtain different positions of employment and so have the need to belong to a different network.

In addition, others may wish to join the network as they learn about its activities. It generally is a good idea to have criteria for membership established by the members well in advance of requests to join the network. In this case, there are no problems in deciding whether or not a person can join the network.

If you're uncertain about who can join, that is, if you don't have membership criteria and the application process well spelled out, potential members may lose interest waiting for you to make up your mind. The number of original members will dwindle and, with no new members added, the network will die rather quickly.

In the event you choose to have membership criteria and application processes, it is essential that they be applied fairly and equally to all potential members. There must be no discrimination either "for" friends or "against" others you may possibly not be willing to have in your network. For this reason, membership matters are generally best resolved by committee action, rather than by one individual.

Some think that membership criteria and application procedures result in an "elitist" network. While this may be true in some instances, if the network is designed for a specific group of individuals, it is necessary to include only those individuals who meet the criteria.

If the membership is open to all interested persons, you probably will have more members than if the membership is restricted to individuals who meet specified criteria. However, if the membership is open to anyone, you may not have the specific focus for the group that was intended when the network was originated. In that case, you may find it necessary to establish subgroups within the network to meet the specific needs of those for whom the network was established.

Once members have joined the network, there must be efforts made to retain them as active, participating members. Participation can be ensured by involving each member in the network activities. Serving on committees, scheduling meetings and being responsible for their conduct, initiating fund-raising projects, and so on, all are activities in which individual members can be involved. If the members aren't active and don't feel that they are a part of the network, they will drop their membership, and the network will suffer.

There must be provision for members to make suggestions to those in leadership roles in the network. Welch recommends that there be a suggestion box where members can offer complaints or suggestions anonymously.[4] Welch asserts that individuals may drop out rather than complain openly about a network that is not meeting their needs.

Meeting Matters

Meetings should be scheduled frequently enough so that matters can be handled in a timely fashion. The membership of the network generally should be responsible for setting the meeting schedule. The network leadership also should have the right to call special meetings of the membership if that is necessary to address a specific issue within a given time frame.

The network meetings can be structured in any manner that best meets the members' needs. The meetings can be "all business," where matters such as membership and other issues are addressed. There can be a combination of social activities, such as a meal or wine and cheese party, followed by business activities. There can be other forms of entertainment, such as plays, choirs, or small musical groups.

Some network groups meet annually for a banquet and dance in addition to their regularly scheduled meetings throughout the year. At that time, spouses of the network members are invited. The evening is primarily devoted to social activities, although there may be such network-related activities as special recognition of members for their accomplishments during the past year.

A business meeting can be combined with a program meeting. In that case, a speaker is engaged to address the group on a topic of interest to them. There can be other educational programs arranged, such as tours, films, other audiovisual shows, displays, exhibits, or demonstrations.

Regardless of how the network meetings are structured, it is important not to lose sight of the purpose for beginning the network. That is, since the network was formed for the purposes of networking, there must be time provided for that activitiy. For that reason, some social time for the members should be built into each meeting time. There can be networking over a meal or over refreshments or during a meeting break.

In order to ensure that networking takes place, at least at initial network meetings, it may be wise to structure small group sessions during the meeting. Individuals are then instructed to join the small group discussing the topic in which they are most interested. An individual with some expertise on the topic may be designated as group leader, in order to avoid the phenomenon of "the blind leading the blind," which may be a reaction of some members to small group activities.

The groups initially may need to be given some questions for discussion in order to provide them with the necessary structure. As the members of the network become more comfortable with one another, and more willing and able to network on their own, the structure provided by the leadership should be reduced.

EVALUATING NETWORK EFFECTIVENESS

In order to continue to be effective in meeting the needs of the membership, there must be some means of evaluating the network on a periodic basis. The entire membership should be involved in the evaluative activities.

A plan to evaluate the network activities is best designed by a small group and then brought to the membership for endorsement or approval.

The composition of the evaluation group should include representation from the leadership of the network as well as members who are not in leadership positions. The group needs to meet only as long as necessary to accomplish its task.

The evaluation task force can get input from the membership as to the kind of evaluation of the network they wish. However, because many of the members may not be able to identify aspects they wish included because of lack of familiarity with evaluation plans, the evaluation task force should be prepared to develop a plan with little or no input from others. It helps if there is an individual with some knowledge about evaluation on the task force, but this is not essential.

The evaluation plan for the network can be simple or complex. A fairly simple evaluation plan can consist of a survey of the members' suggestions for improvement of the network. The survey can be conducted in writing, whereby an instrument is designed and circulated to the membership. The instrument can be constructed to contain four questions:

- What do you like about this network?
- What do you dislike about this network?
- What would you do differently if you were "in charge" of this network?
- What else would you like to see accomplished in this network?

The responses to these questions can be collated by the evaluation task force and then presented to the membership for discussion and resolution of the issues raised. Or, the evaluation task force can review the responses and make recommendations to the membership for improvements in the network.

If the network members are comfortable enough with one another and the evaluation process, they can discuss these questions in small groups. A leader and recorder should be assigned for each group or selected by the group members. The leader is responsible for facilitating the discussion and keeping the group on the topic at hand. The recorder is responsible for writing down the essence of the group discussion. These group reports then are given to the evaluation task force for follow-up and are presented to the leadership of the network or to the membership at large for subsequent action.

A more complex but highly effective evaluation plan is an adaptation of the transactional evaluation process as described by Rippey.[5] In this method of evaluation, network members are asked to write anonymously three problems they perceive with the network. The information is then sent to an individual for tabulating. Preferably, this individual should be someone other than a member of the network in order that the person not be able to identify the originator.

The individual who receives the members' surveys then tabulates the problems identified. Some patterns should emerge as several members identify the same or similar problems. The problems that most of the members of the network identify then are arrayed in the form of a questionnaire. The questionnaire should contain between 20 and 25 items.

Each of the items should be stated exactly as the member stated it, if possible. Problems that are similar in nature should be stated as closely as possible to one member's original statement. Minor grammatical changes or modifications can be made by the person developing the questionnaire, but that person should be cautious not to distort the meaning of the individual's statement or to make it unrecognizable to the individual who initially wrote the statement.

The purpose of this step is to enable members to recognize their contributions to the evaluation process. Several of the members will note that what they said was quoted as a questionnaire item. In this way, the evaluation becomes "theirs" rather than an outsider's.

After the items are listed on a questionnaire, a rating scale is added. The rating scale should allow the persons responding to indicate whether they strongly agree with the statement, agree with the statement, are neutral (neither agree nor disagree with the statement), disagree with the statement, or strongly disagree with the statement.

Once the items and rating scale are arrayed on the form, the questionnaire is sent to all members of the network. Each person is asked to complete the rating of the identified problems of the network and mail the completed form to the same individual who designed the rating form.

It generally is a good idea to establish a deadline for return of the forms. From two to three weeks is ample time to allow for the forms to be completed and returned.

To reduce the costs of the evaluation process, the questionnaires can be distributed at a network meeting. There must be ample time allotted for each member to complete the questionnaire during the meeting. Avoid allowing only a few minutes at the end of the meeting for questionnaire completion; members will be eager to leave and probably will not devote the time necessary to do a careful job. The results of the evaluation may then be biased because of the manner in which the forms were completed.

The same person who designed the questionnaire receives the forms that were returned by mail or completed at a network meeting and then tabulates the ratings, indicating how many members agreed with or disagreed with the problem statements. The results of the tabulations then are presented to the membership for discussion.

By using this method of evaluation, the problem of people dropping out of an organization rather than complaining in front of the entire group will be circumvented. All members of the group now have had their attention focused on the problems in the system. The problems identified are now a group concern rather than an individual one.

At the time the problems of the network are discussed there must be an individual skilled in group process to lead the discussion. The group should be encouraged to openly discuss the ratings of the problems, particularly those with which the majority of the members strongly agreed.

Because of the intimate nature of some of the problems that have been identified, it may be uncomfortable for some individuals in the group. For example, it may be difficult for the network leadership to take responsibility for some of the network's problems even if the results of the questionnaire tabulations indicate that they were responsible. The group leader must assist the members to discuss the problems with the leaders in a nonthreatening way that will lead to some constructive action toward resolution of the identified problems.

The discussion leader must encourage all those present to be open and honest. This is essential if the evaluative process is to be of assistance in the growth and development of the network.

The evaluation of a network is an integral component of the ongoing process of establishing and maintaining the network. If the network is to survive, it has to be responsive to the needs of its members and function in a worthwhile manner. Evaluation, whether planned simply or using a more elaborate design, will be of assistance in determining the effectiveness of your network.

SUMMARY

Networks have been effective for women of all ages and in all walks of life. There already are networks that respond to the many and varied needs of women in their personal and professional lives. Despite the existence of these networks, however, there may be situations in which an individual wishes to start a network of his or her own.

When one individual has a need for a network, it probably is a fair assumption that there are others who would be interested in and benefit from that same network as well. When these individuals come together with their similar needs and interests, starting a new network is the logical next step. Starting a network requires only that the individuals be interested and determined that a new network should exist.

The steps to follow in starting new networks are simple and will help to ensure that the networks succeed. Involvement and commitment of the network membership will ensure that the new network is effective in meeting members' needs. Long-range planning and ongoing evaluation will ensure that the network is long lived.

NOTES

1. Mary Scott Welch, *Networking* (New York: Harcourt Brace Jovanovich, 1980), p. 147.
2. Ibid., p. 232.
3. J. William Pfeiffer and John E. Jones, "Who Am I?: A Cocktail Mix," *A Handbook of Structured Experiences for Human Relations Training,* vol. 1 (Iowa City, Iowa: University Associates, 1969), pp. 19–20.
4. Welch, *Networking,* p. 236.
5. R. M. Rippey, ed., *Studies in Transactional Evaluation* (Berkeley, Calif.; McCutchan, 1973), pp. 1-23.

Chapter 4

Mentoring

Mentoring, like networking, has primarily been the preserve of men. *Webster's New Collegiate Dictionary* defines a mentor as "a trusted counselor or guide." One excellent example of men's mentoring was the relationship between Merlyn and the young King Arthur, graphically depicted in the movie *Camelot*. Other examples of mentoring appear in history, in such diverse areas as sports, business, and the arts.

MENTORS FOR MEN

Mentors are viewed by many as the key to success in the business world. In an article in the *Harvard Business Review*, editors Eliza G. C. Collins and Patricia Scott described a series of interviews they conducted with executives of the Jewel Companies.[1] In those interviews three executives discussed their mentor relationships. Each identified someone in his background with the corporation who had assisted him in achieving success within the company. Generally, that individual held a higher position in the corporate structure than did the protégé, or person being guided. Each stated that he would not have been as successful if it had not been for his mentor.

The mentors revealed that they did not necessarily expect the person being mentored to replace them when they left the company or retired, although one indicated that his protégé "hadn't been here too long before I knew he was my successor." Though all three expected their protégés to get ahead in the company, none viewed the protégé's success as any personal threat to themselves.

All three executives stated that the relationship between them and the individual they mentored was not based on treating the protégé as a "fair haired boy." In each instance, the mentor clearly identified the protégé's competence in doing the job that needed to be done. One mentor stated that he wouldn't have done as much as he had for his protégé if "he didn't have it, in my judgment."

This series of interviews illustrates the role of mentors as individuals who "grease the skids," who advise, counsel, and teach. In a typical mentor relationship, an older, well-established man in a business or corporation will seek out a younger man who has some promise. The older man generally is well established in the business and has risen to the top of the corporate ladder. He is now quite successful, and so seeks to pass some of his knowledge and skills on to another individual in the company.

Typically, the young man will be bright, articulate, and grateful for this helping hand on his way up to the top. The young person learns from the older person's experiences. His mentor will offer advice on such diverse matters as who to get to know in the company, what clothes to wear, and what clubs or business and professional groups to join. The young man will be introduced to significant others by his mentor. He will be invited to all the important company meetings. His mentor can be counted on to drop his name at the appropriate moment in all the most advantageous situations.

Mentorship, in this example, goes beyond the older man's serving as a role model for the younger man. Mentorship in the business world implies active participation in the relationship, a willingness to assist another individual to get ahead.

To determine whether mentor relationships actually were effective in the development of corporation executives, Gerard R. Roche, president and chief executive officer of a consulting firm that deals with executive selection, conducted a study of executives that included questions about relationships between mentors and protégés.[2] The study results showed that these relationships were fairly prevalent in the business world, but that not every executive had a mentor. The study also revealed that the mentor relationship has become more prevalent within the last twenty years.

Roche concluded that executives who had had a mentor "earn more money at a younger age, are better educated, are more likely to follow a career plan, and, in turn, sponsor more protégés than executives who have not had a mentor."[3]

While most mentor relationships are confined to the work situation, it is not inconceivable that a typical men's mentor relationship might even extend into both individuals' personal lives. The young man and his mentor might play tennis or golf together. The mentor might invite the young man (and his wife) for dinner or an evening's entertainment at the country club.

The mentorship can begin on a formal basis, such as when the older man is assigned to "orient" the younger man to the company or the young man is involved in an "internship" or "apprenticeship" in the corporation. In two of the instances described by the three Jewel Companies executives, the mentor relationship began because the mentor was administratively responsible for supervising the protégé. In the third instance, the protégé was a subordinate of the mentor and was selected for sponsorship because the mentor noted the protégé's skills, abilities, and potential.

The mentor relationship can begin in a less formal manner, such as when the vice-president says, "Young man, I like your style." In one instance, a Jewel Companies executive told how he was "chosen" by his mentor. The protégé described knowing his mentor as the father of a university classmate. The mentor recommended the individual for an important position in the company. Both mentor and protégé subsequently worked together for years.

These typical examples of mentorship of males by other men illustrates how mentor relationships contribute to the old boys' network, as the "young boys" are brought along to replace the "old boys." Indeed, each of three Jewel Companies executives served as a mentor to his successor. These mentor relationships between three successive chief executives "have played an important role in shaping the organization."[4]

MENTORS FOR WOMEN

That mentorship is crucial for women's success has been recognized by Gail Sheehy, author of the popular book *Passages,* on stages of adult development. Sheehy states that "The lack of mentors. . . . is a great developmental handicap."[5]

The first women who began to rise to high positions in corporations became acutely aware of the mentoring phenomenon but observed that mentoring was reserved for the male employees. Most of these first successful businesswomen did not have mentors to assist them.

In general, women in business have experienced mentoring relationships much more often than have men, according to the findings of Roche's study. Those women who responded to Roche's questionnaire all indicated that they had had a mentor and most of them reported having more mentors than had men. Women reported having three mentors and men two. The women also had female mentors more often than did the men, although the majority of mentors for both women and men were men.

In some instances now, women in business are aggressively seeking out mentors in their employment settings in order to take advantage of the benefits that men have received from such relationships in the past. Margaret Hennig and Anne Jardim, authors of *The Managerial Woman,* describe how fatherlike (male) sponsors are necessary for women, particularly those without family business connections, to reach top management positions.[6]

Problems can arise, however, when women seek out mentors in business, as most individuals highly placed in large corporations are men. This creates difficulty when an executive wishes to serve as mentor for an up-and-coming young woman. There often may be misperception by others about their relationship. The attribution of a personal relationship where none may actually exist can be harmful, both personally and professionally, to both parties.

MENTORS IN NURSING

In the early stages of their professional careers, young nurses often establish relationships with their teachers, counselors, or perhaps the head nurse or supervisor on the nursing units in their first clinical practice or employment setting. The young nurse looks to this individual for support and advice. Though these relationships often are helpful for the nurse during the time they exist, they generally are fairly transient relationships. As the nurse moves on to other clinical practice areas or to other employment settings, the relationship is terminated. These relationships may not be classified as mentoring relationships, but are more instances in which the young nurse patterns behaviors of his or her role model.

By and large, mentorship has not occurred to a great extent in the nursing profession. Lucie Kelly, noted nurse leader and author of *Dimensions of Professional Nursing,* describes the mentor system that is critically needed in the nursing profession as "a formal or informal system between a prestigious, established older person and a younger one, wherein the older guides, counsels and critiques the younger, teaching him/her survival and advancement in a certain field or profession."[7] Although Kelly describes a one-to-one mentor relationship, a person can "mentor" more than one protégé, and a protégé can have more than one mentor.

Mentors are needed in nursing to ensure that the heritage of the profession is passed on from generation to generation. Mentors also are needed to ensure that nursing leaders will emerge from the nurses who are beginning their careers in the profession.

Kathleen May, Afaf Meleis, and Patricia Winstead-Fry, writing in *Nursing Outlook,*[8] described mentorship of young scholars in nursing, indicating the potential that mentorship might have in the development of scholarliness in nursing. While the relationship of sponsorship to scholarliness has not yet been empirically tested, the authors suggest that mentorship may have an influence on the development of teachers, clinicians, and administrators in nursing. They further state that "nurses are becoming increasingly interested in the phenomenon of mentorship as they seek to identify the resources that can aid in professional development and achievement."[9]

Some instances of nurses' interest and activity in mentorship have appeared in the nursing literature. In her doctoral dissertation titled "A Group Profile of Contemporary Influentials in American Nursing," Connie Vance found that 83 percent of known nursing leaders reported having mentors in their professional lives. Of these nursing leaders, 93 percent reported that they were serving as mentors to others, most often students in their academic programs.[10]

In an article about her firsthand experiences in a mentor relationship, Patty Hawken describes an apprenticeship of a year's duration in which she served as an administrative associate to the dean of a school of nursing in order to learn the various aspects of nursing education administration. She relates that the experience, under the mentorship of the dean, was "so worthwhile that it encouraged me to provide a similar opportunity for others."[11]

In another instance, Barbara Ann Larson conducted a study to explore the relationship of job satisfaction of the nursing leaders in hospital settings who had a mentor relationship with the job satisfaction of those who had not had a mentor relationship.[12] The relationship was measured by means of a standardized instrument and a questionnaire about mentor relationships and the nurse's career choice.

Most of those responding to the questionnaire indicated that nursing had been their first career choice. Overall, these nursing leaders' responses indicated satisfaction with their jobs. The measurement of job satisfaction encompassed several variables, among them (1) opportunities for promotion, (2) supervision, (3) pay, and (4) co-workers.

A majority of those nursing leaders in hospital settings who responded to the questionnaire reported having had a mentor. The job satisfaction scores for those nurses who had mentors was higher than the job satisfaction scores for nurses who reported not having mentors. Those nurses who reported being mentors for others also reported higher job satisfaction.

Not all nurses are willing, or able, to serve as mentors, just as not all nurses will be willing to be mentored. Some nurses may choose a nurse mentor; others may choose a mentor from outside the profession of nursing. What is needed is for nurses to become aware of the process of mentoring and what is involved on both sides of the relationship so that they can make intelligent decisions about the role they wish to play in a mentor relationship.

WHEN MENTORING OCCURS

The study by Roche revealed that mentor relationships can begin at any point in an individual's life. Typically, for men, the mentor relationship began during college, during military service, or during the first five years of their careers, with the next most frequent period for the establishment of mentor relationships being during the sixth to tenth years. After that period of time, the need for a sponsor seems to be less acute. By the time a man has been active in his career for over ten years, he is not likely to be willing or able to accept a mentor relationship. Also, at that point in a man's career, he most likely has already achieved a level of success.

In contrast, women formed their mentor relationships during the sixth to tenth years of their careers. Roche concludes that this finding results from women deciding at that point in time that they have careers instead of merely "work."

Most of the nursing leaders in Larson's study had been employed in nursing for over ten years. They had held their present positions for periods of time ranging from two to five years. The time period during which they established their mentor relationships was not indicated.

The three executives from Jewel Companies did not describe the time period in their careers during which they established their mentor relationships. One said that he was "only 25" when he was recommended for a position with the company by his mentor; there was, however, no indication of how many years prior to that he had begun work in his chosen field.

WHO MENTORS

In the Jewel Companies example, it is apparent that the chief executive officer of the corporation was the mentor. While each of the three executives indicated that he mentored his successor, each also stated they had mentored others in the company.

The respondents, both male and female, in the Roche study, identified as their mentors primarily their department or division heads or their immediate supervisors. Mentors also were presidents or chief executive officers of the corporation, but to a lesser extent. Professors and teachers also served as mentors. Almost the same number of respondents identified friends as their mentors. Relatives and those classified in a category of

"Other" were reported to be their mentors by similar numbers of respondents.

The relationship of mentors to nurse leaders in the study conducted by Larson was primarily supervisory. The majority of mentors occupied such positions as supervisor or assistant or associate director of nursing. Mentors frequently were in positions in nursing education, such as a teacher, professor, or academic advisor. And, other frequently reported mentors were the nurses' colleagues. These nurse leaders reported few mentors among friends or family, and even fewer in other categories, such as ministers or others outside the field of nursing.

When friends were indicated as the nurse leaders' mentors, it was because the friend currently was in a similar situation or had previously been in such a situation. In the former instance, the friends would support each other as they shared similar experiences. In the latter instance, the mentor would most likely be trying to help his or her friend avoid making similar mistakes. Thus, the friend could benefit from the mentor's previous experiences.

Mentors described by Vance also tended to occupy administrative positions. More respondents from the population Vance studied identified teachers and professional work colleagues as their mentors than did the nurses whom Larson studied.

THE ROLE OF THE MENTOR

Traditionally, men serving as mentors for other men have been successful in their own right. They are educationally and experientially prepared for their positions, and have achieved some amount of success. Freed from the stress of seeking ever higher positions on the corporate ladder, they are able to devote time and energy to helping others achieve some of the same success they have already attained.

The mentor has to be willing to expend energy on the relationship. The mentor advises and counsels the individual on both personal and professional matters. In effect, the mentor assumes a fair degree of responsibility for the career advancement of the person being mentored. The mentor provides the opportunities; the individual being mentored then has to take advantage of those opportunities. If the person being mentored doesn't succeed, the "fault" may be with the mentor as much as with the person being mentored.

Some of the characteristics necessary for the mentor to possess if the mentor relationship is to be successful include:

- good interpersonal relationships

- self-confidence
- willingness to share

The mentor must have good interpersonal relations skills. The mentoring relationship involves trust and intimacy between the two individuals. The mentor may learn information about the individual he or she is mentoring that must be kept in confidence. The person being mentored must trust his or her mentor with that information. Some degree of intimacy is necessary if the relationship is to be successful in helping the person being mentored. Both individuals in the relationship have to be comfortable with each other.

Mentors also have to have good interpersonal relationships with others. If the mentor is to introduce the protégé to other influentials, the mentor has to have established good relationships with those people. If good relationships with others don't already exist, these individuals are not likely to accept a mentor's recommendation.

The mentor has to be confident about his or her ability to help others succeed. The necessity for this self-confidence, perhaps, explains why most mentors already are successful individuals. They generally occupy positions of authority in the institutions in which they work. They know the organizations in which they are employed. Because they have the confidence that comes from already having made it, they are more likely to be able to help others make it, too.

Mentors have to be individuals who deserve respect because of their professional capability and personal characteristics. They usually have the respect of their colleagues and peers, both inside and outside of their employing agency. Some of that respect may be attributed to the mentor's position, but it also should be based on the mentor's competence.

It is not necessary that the person being mentored "like" the mentor. Because of the intimacy of the relationship, however, it is helpful if the mentor is liked as well as admired.

Mentor relationships, according to the results of the Roche study, often develop into lengthy friendships. Nearly half of those individuals who reported having mentors indicated at the time of the study that they had maintained their relationships with their mentors. Even though the mentor relationship was, in some instances, not described as a friendship, most individuals reported that the relationship was "friendly" or "close."

Of those who related that they had not maintained their relationship with their mentor, most reported that the relationship had lasted for a long period of time. Four of every ten mentor relationships lasted ten or more years, and three in ten were maintained for a period of from five to nine years.[13]

The mentor has to be willing and able to spend time with the person being mentored. That means the mentor has to have a personal interest in the individual and be capable of putting that interest into constructive action. If the mentor is overcommitted, and unable to devote the necessary time to the person being mentored, it is unlikely that much will be gained from the relationship.

The mentor has to enter the relationship with a view toward giving rather than getting satisfaction from the relationship. The mentor has to be willing to share his or her knowledge and experiences with the person being mentored. Although tremendously ego lifting, the mentoring relationship primarily is for the benefit of the person being mentored rather than for the gratification of the mentor. The mentor must be able to contribute to the growth and development of another person without simultaneously seeking enhancement of his or her own development. Often such growth, and certainly much satisfaction, are serendipitous effects of a mentoring relationship, but they are not the primary purpose.

The mentor also has specific functions, as defined by Levinson in his book *The Seasons of a Man's Life*.[14] Levinson defined the roles of the mentor as:

- a teacher
- a sponsor
- a host
- an exemplar
- a counselor

Mentor as Teacher

Acting as a teacher is the generally perceived role of the mentor. Since most mentor relationships begin when the protégé is in the initial learning and growing period of a career, it is natural that the mentor would be expected to be a teacher. Since most mentors also are at a position above that of their protégé, they would convey their experiences, thus teaching the protégé the best way of doing things. Levinson identified the mentor's purpose as a teacher to enhance the protégé's skills and to further his or her intellectual development.

A nurse in an administrative role in a hospital who assists his or her subordinate in developing leadership skills is acting as a teacher in the mentor relationship. The faculty person in the school of nursing who encourages a student to rewrite a term paper for publication, then describes the process of manuscript publication, also is acting as a mentor/teacher.

The mentor relationship, because of the emphasis on its tutorial nature, should be a natural occurrence in teaching/learning situations.

Mentor as Sponsor

Mentors also serve as protégés' sponsors. In this role, the mentor assists the protégé to obtain professional opportunities to which he or she might not otherwise have access. Sponsors ease the protégé's way in the work world. The mentor as sponsor smooths the path up the ladder of success.

In this role, the nurse leader, knowing of a younger nurse's interest in writing for publication, might introduce the younger nurse to an editor or publisher. The mentor also may provide a protégé with an opportunity to collaborate on a project with him or her, sharing the credit and giving the protégé visibility.

Mentor as Host

Acting as a host, the mentor introduces the protégé to the culture and customs of the occupation. Here, the mentor may caution the protégé about the appropriate way to dress. For example, the mentor might say "At the opening night reception at the conference, you may wish to wear a cocktail dress. For the business and program sessions, a suit or a dress with a jacket is appropriate. Hardly anyone wears pants to these meetings any more." Thus, the mentor transmits the expectations of the group to the protégé.

The mentor arranges for the protégé to become acquainted with "significant" others in the organization. These important people may have some influence over the protégé's ability to succeed in the corporation. Because of longevity or position in the corporation, the mentor is in a position to be certain that the person being mentored knows all of the right people. Introductions to such individuals are more easily accomplished through a mentor.

Examples of this mentor role occur daily, as nurses new to organizations or agencies are introduced to those others with whom they must work. There hardly is an orientation in a nurse's new employment setting that doesn't contain some words about "who's to know" in that setting. Along with identifying who the newly employed nurse should know, there generally are some words of caution; those individuals the nurse would do well to stay away from are identified as well.

Mentor as Exemplar

The exemplar role is filled by the mentor when acting as a role model for the protégé. The mentor serves as a personal example of ways in which the protégé should act. Such role modeling can be conscious and deliberate, such as when the mentor says "Now I want you to watch how I conduct this meeting. Then, we'll talk about some of what I did that was helpful in facilitating group process and decision making."

Mentors' role modeling also can be an unconscious act. Faculty members in basic educational programs in nursing, particularly those who are involved in students' clinical experiences, are in key positions to serve as exemplars.

Mentor as Counselor

The mentor acts as a counselor when he or she provides support, advice, and feedback to the protégé. In this role, the mentor combines the activities of teacher and exemplar, coaching the protégé into appropriate forms of behavior as well as actually demonstrating them.

In an example of a mentor in this role, a nurse might tell a colleague "If I were you, I'd approach the director with several options rather than only one. She doesn't like to be handed what she considers an ultimatum. Are there alternatives other than just the one you're now considering?" Or "It might be more helpful if you start the patient care plan meeting by asking the aides what they know about the patient's illness. Once you know where they are in relation to understanding the patient's illness, you can build on what they already are familiar with when you work together on a care plan."

The mentor performs the various functions and responsibilities of the role at different times in the mentor relationship. There is considerable overlap in the functions, and, of course, not every mentor will possess the necessary characteristics to the same degree. Nonetheless, serving as a mentor carries with it certain specific responsibilities.

THE ROLE OF THE PERSON BEING MENTORED

The person being mentored also has responsibilities that must be met to ensure the success of the mentoring relationship. This individual also must actively participate in the mentor relationship.

The mentor relationship as described here implies active roles and ongoing participation for both the mentor and the protégé. Mentoring, in this sense, goes beyond the traditional role model or preceptor concept.

While role modeling is an effective way of learning, it may result from a passive relationship between an older, more experienced person and a young one. In many instances, young graduate nurses model behaviors that they have seen their teachers or head nurses perform. The younger nurse may unintentionally model some behaviors that are ineffective but that he or she learned and is doing by rote, rather than understanding the reasons for the behavior.

Preceptor relationships generally involve both parties more actively. In a preceptor relationship, one individual teaches, supervises, or coaches the other. Preceptor relationships can become mentor relationships, but they also can be quite limited in their scope and depth.

For example, a preceptor relationship established between a new graduate nurse upon her first employment in a hospital setting and a head nurse may encompass only "orientation." The preceptor may be interested in the new nurse and be willing to assist in any way possible to acquaint him or her with the working situation, but may take no further interest in the nurse's career development beyond this specific employment. The preceptor may spend a considerable amount of time with the new nurse, but when the nurse is assigned to a different nursing unit or shift, the relationship may terminate.

In order to engage in a satisfying mentoring relationship, it helps if both parties know that the relationship exists. Then they can both take active parts in maintaining the relationship for their mutual benefit. If a young nurse seeks out a mentor, he or she is in a better position to explain what it is he or she hopes to gain from the relationship, rather than copying behaviors at random, hoping that some of the behaviors learned will be effective in helping him or her succeed.

The young nurse has to be at a point in his or her career where a mentor will be helpful. Judging by the results of the Roche study, the most appropriate time for a nurse to have a mentor may be early in his or her career.

The point in the nurse's career at which the mentor is chosen also will influence the selection of the individual who could become the nurse's mentor. If the nurse hasn't yet completed his or her basic educational preparation for nursing, for example, a nursing leader who is well-known in the field may be less appropriate as a mentor than a nurse faculty member or the student's counselor. By contrast, if a nurse has become fairly successful in a field of practice, a mentor may not be able to do more than the nurse can alone.

The person being mentored must be willing to learn from his or her mentor. The individual has to be able to accept feedback, whether positive or negative, and be able to use it constructively.

The person being mentored has to be capable of initiating and maintaining an intimate adult relationship, which requires a certain amount of maturity. The relationship is between an older and a younger person, and should not be similar to hero worship or having an adolescent crush. Neither is the relationship one of collegiality, at least at its beginning. The person being mentored has to recognize the parameters of the relationship and be careful not to violate them to the detriment of the existing relationship with the mentor and others that may follow.

Finally, the person being mentored has an obligation to assist others in turn, when he or she is in a position to become a mentor. Roche identified the tendency for those who were mentored to serve as mentors. The nurse leaders in Larson's study reported they were more likely to serve as mentors if they had had a mentor themselves. If they had not had a mentor, then they were not likely to serve as a mentor to others. It is only through providing opportunities for others in the same manner that similar opportunities were provided for us that we will make mentoring an integral part of the nursing profession.

ESTABLISHING A MENTOR RELATIONSHIP

The mentor relationship is a specific type of helping relationship. Those who seek help tend to seek it from those in a position to provide the help needed. For this reason, then, nurse mentors generally are in administrative positions.

Vance describes the mentor relationship as having characteristics in common with the relationship of the parent with the child.[15] Some of the characteristics of the mentor relationship, however, differ strikingly from the parent/child relationship. The successful mentor relationship requires maturity and independence on the part of the person being mentored. In the event that the mentor relationship begins to closely approximate the parental relationship, to the point where it no longer is conducive to the individual's personal and professional growth, then the relationship will not be successful, and may even be damaging to one or both parties.

Formal Mentor Relationships

Some of these mentor relationships are established in a formal manner, such as when executives in the Jewel Companies are assigned to look after a person who is new to the company. In nursing, someone generally is assigned to look after a new graduate or new nursing employee on a nursing unit. Occasionally, the person assigned to the new employee is from the hospital's staff development or other educational department.

Formal establishment of mentor relationships is not encouraged to any great extent in the health care professions. Some hospitals are beginning to encourage "internships" or "preceptorships" for new graduates, newly employed nurses, or those who are returning to practice after extended periods of professional inactivity. Such practices certainly are innovative, but as yet are not widespread.

In the event that a formal relationship is established, either one of the parties can initiate the mentor relationship. The individual serving as mentor may recognize the protégé's potential and wish to assist in that person's career development. The protégé may realize that the other individual has knowledge and skills to convey, and so may wish to take full advantage of the opportunity to learn and grow professionally.

Because of the identified need for information and support of women in their career development, some networks have as one of their purposes facilitating mentor relationships. The explicit matching of network contacts as partners is a formalized method of establishing a mentor relationship.

Informal Mentor Relationships

Mentor relationships also can be established more informally. In such cases, for example, a young nurse or new employee makes friends with someone by choice rather than by assignment. While this relationship is primarily that of friendship, there also can be elements of the mentor relationship included.

Informal mentor relationships are established by the mentor or by the protégé. In the former case, the mentor initiates the establishment of the sponsorship, taking the protégé "under his or her wing," as it were. Most mentor relationships begin with the mentor's identifying someone who has potential and initiating a helping relationship.

In some instances, however, if the nurse finds that he or she is not being "discovered" by someone who wishes to serve as his or her mentor, it may be necessary to ask someone to be a mentor. The protégé may begin by seeking advice or counsel from the more experienced person. It may be difficult to ask a person to be a mentor, so the relationship might start with the nurse's asking for feedback on a manuscript or advice on a dissertation topic. Subsequent contacts can be made in the same informal fashion, with the end result being a mentor relationship.

Using networking skills is essential in establishing a relationship with a potential mentor. You must prepare yourself so that you can benefit from the mentor relationship. You must also present yourself well so that you appear to be someone worth the mentor's investment of time and energy.

As nurses, and other women as well, become more aware of the need for and the value of, the mentor relationship, such relationships should increase in frequency. At that time, too, it should be easier to establish a mentor relationship because the "rules" will be better known. At the present time, most of the literature on the subject indicates that it is the mentor who selects the person to mentor. But, rather than suffer from the lack of a mentor relationship, it would be better to take the necessary risks to initiate a mentor relationship on your own.

Mentor relationships occur naturally in most instances. There is no formal declaration that the mentor is acting as a mentor, nor does the protégé necessarily make a formal statement that he or she is filling that role. The Jewel Companies executives stated that they were consciously trying to develop their protégés, but the protégés were not able, in all instances, to perceive that they were being "developed." Since the mentor relationship is so often established on an informal basis and evolves gradually, it may be only in retrospect that each is able to identify the role he or she played in the mentor relationship. As nurses become more aware of the value of mentor relationships, they may very well formalize such roles to a greater extent.

BENEFITS OF MENTORSHIP

The benefits of a mentor relationship are similar to the benefits of networking. A mentor relationship can provide opportunities for professional growth and achievement that might otherwise not have existed.

Among the most commonly identified benefits of a mentor relationship are:

- career planning
- leadership development
- personal satisfaction

Career Planning

One significant benefit of the mentor relationship identified by the respondents in the Roche study was assistance with career planning. They also revealed that mentors had less influence over them personally than over their careers. Most of the respondents reported that their mentors had had a substantial influence on their careers. Considerably fewer related that the influence of their mentors was "average," and even less identified that influence as "extraordinary."[16]

Roche provides more specific information about the benefits of the mentor relationship related to the career planning aspects than do many other writers on the topic. For example, those respondents in the Roche study who reported having had a mentor were younger than those who did not have a mentor, but they were financially compensated better. They also reported increases in salaries that were higher than their counterparts who had not had mentors. There was no appreciable difference reported in perquisites between the two groups.

Those who had mentors were better educated than those who did not. Roche postulates that "It seems likely that the better educated young executive 'on the way up' more frequently either attracts the attention of a superior, or being more appreciative of the value of a sponsor, initiates a relationship."[17] The study results, however, did not reveal at what point in the mentor relationship those individuals had obtained their advanced education. Here, Roche apparently does not consider that the mentor may have influenced the protégé to obtain additional education in order to advance more rapidly.

The Jewel Companies executives also discussed career planning as an important part of their mentor relationships. The career planning aspect was present in the relationship whether the executive was in the role of mentor or in the role of protégé.

The mentors of the influential nurses studied by Vance provided assistance to those nurses in areas that were categorized as "(1) career advice, guidance, promotion, (2) professional role modeling, (3) intellectual and scholarly stimulation, (4) inspiration and idealism, (5) teaching, advising, tutoring, (6) emotional support, and (7) other."[18] In the "other" category were such areas of help as financial advice and sharing. The areas of help received by these influential nurses from their mentors coincided with the functions of mentors identified by Levinson (mentors as teachers, role models, and counselors).

Leadership Development

Mentors also act to motivate their protégés, encouraging them to perform activities they might not otherwise attempt. Several of the respondents studied by Vance stated that their mentors had encouraged them to make speeches and write for publication. Particularly in the area of writing for publication in the nursing literature, for example, can a mentor be of assistance to a protégé. There is little content related to writing for publication in most nursing education programs. Papers produced in baccalaureate or graduate nursing programs, such as term papers or theses, are not appropriate for publication in their existing form. Nurses may avail themselves of one of the myriad courses on how to write, but the general result of attendance at such a learning activity is the knowledge of how to write but not the skills to actually write. With a mentor, particularly one who has published successfully, the nurse has an expert who can provide assistance in the form of counsel, advice, and support, over the entire writing process from generating the idea to submitting the manuscript.

Giving speeches and writing for publication are only two of the leadership activities that can be developed through the mentor relationship. Hawken's description of her experiences as a protégé to a dean is an excellent example of a mentor's leadership development activities.[19]

Another leadership skill that can be transmitted through the mentor relationship is that of creativity. Mentors can demonstrate unique and creative solutions to the problems they encounter, thus modeling appropriate behaviors for the protégé. Creativity can be reinforced and rewarded by the mentor.

If the protégé has an audience for his or her creativity that will be at the same time supportive and challenging, he or she will be more likely to experiment a bit. Mentors can assist protégés to take risks by encouraging the dissemination of new ideas and by supporting their protégés during the period when their new ideas are being tested by professional colleagues.

By their mentoring activities, mentors perform leadership functions in their profession. In a small way, and possibly in a larger sense, they may influence the direction of the profession by developing the profession's future leaders.

Personal Satisfaction

Both the mentor and the protégé can benefit from the personal satisfaction that results from a mentor relationship. This personal satisfaction extends over the life of the relationship and beyond.

For the mentor the satisfaction primarily comes from knowing he or she has helped someone grow and mature, both professionally and personally. Mentorship provides a sense of having done something worthwhile. Watching the development of an individual whom you have assisted is closely akin to raising a child. The rewards often are intangible for mentors as for parents.

Protégés often continue to use aspects of networking in the mentor relationship. They "report" to their mentors about their current activities, what they are involved in, and what their plans are. In this way, the relationship is ongoing, even though the mentor may have little influence once the protégé is successfully "launched."

Whether the mentorship occurs over the course of an entire relationship or only occasionally, mentoring has benefits for the mentor. Being asked to review a manuscript for publication, for example, and then seeing the manuscript in print gives an individual personal satisfaction.

Serving as a mentor is an "ego trip." A mentor enjoys being asked for advice and assistance and being involved in decision making. Whether on an ongoing basis with one individual or sporadically with many individuals, the mentor receives positive feedback for his or her efforts. This feedback can take the form of seeing a finished product, such as a manuscript published or a speech given, or it can be in hearing reports from the protégé or others about the protégé's success.

Being involved with protégés keeps the mentor on the crest of the state of the art, in touch with new ideas and fresh insights, for the protégé has much to offer the mentor, particularly the opportunity to perfect his or her mentoring. For the protégé, there is tremendous satisfaction in the mentor relationship that may be more tangible than the satisfaction gained by the mentor. The protégé benefits from the visible effects of career planning and leadership development. The mentor "opens doors" for the protégé and provides professional opportunities to advance from which the protégé can derive much satisfaction. Roche described the satisfaction of those individuals who had had mentors as much greater than those who had not had mentors.[20]

PROBLEMS OF THE MENTOR RELATIONSHIP

Although there are distinct and significant benefits in mentor relationships, there also can be problems. Some of these problems are directly related to the participants in the relationship, while others relate to the characteristics of the mentor relationship itself.

There are problems with the participants in a mentor relationship when both are women. Traditionally, women are socialized to expect others (particularly males) to support them. In the mentor relationship, the mentor provides support for others. While, as we have noted, there are benefits that accrue for the mentor in the relationship, the primary focus of support and help is on the protégé.

Most women also have been raised to believe that their careers are not an integral part of their lives. According to Hennig and Jardim, "Men expressly relate the jobs they do to their concept of career as advancement, as upward progression. . . . . Women separate the two issues completely: a job is in the here and now and a career is an intensely personal goal . . . . .''21

Many women, including nurses, see their work as a "job" that primarily ensures their earning a living. By contrast, men view their employment as a series of tasks to be completed, as a way of life, and as a means of support. Women, then, tend to view their employment as temporary and short term, with an end in sight when they no longer have to support themselves but can rely on someone else to support them. Men view their career as a long-term situation, as they have been raised to believe they must always support not only themselves but their families as well.

When women serve as mentors, then, they may have difficulty assisting a protégé with career planning. Protégés, as well, may have difficulty being responsive to a mentor who has as a primary purpose career guidance for them. Without the emphasis of career necessity that men possess, it is difficult for women, whether mentors or protégés, to focus on career development as the primary benefit of the mentor relationship.

Women also have learned that other women are primarily in competition with them (usually for males). Because the mentor relationship requires an intense emotional involvement for both (something women have traditionally reserved for their relationships with men), it has been difficult for women to serve as mentors or as protégés of other women. Mentors may have difficulty with the success of the protégé, particularly if the protégé's success is perceived as being a threat to the mentor.

Another problem related to mentor relationships when both parties are women is that there are so few women (and nurses) in positions of power and influence who can serve as mentors. The influential nurses studied by Vance reported that they served as mentors to other nurses, but the population of influential nurses included only 71 individuals.

The lack of female mentors for women in business has been repeatedly identified. Many of the women who occupy positions in corporations often describe their success as attributable to "luck" or "being in the right place at the right time." These women often don't see the need to serve as mentors to other women. Then, too, many of these women are still in a position where they are uncertain about their own employment status and so lack the necessary time and energy to devote to a mentor relationship.

In addition, many nurses do not perceive themselves as successful and, thus, do not have the self-confidence to serve as mentors for someone else. Even nurses who are perceived by others as being quite successful in the profession may not share that perception.

This lack of self-esteem is apparent in the protégé role as well as in the mentor role. Many women feel it is unfair to ask for help unless they can offer something in return. Because of this, nurses may be reluctant to ask for assistance, thinking they do not deserve to receive it.

These and other attributes of women create difficulties for the establishment and maintenance of a successful mentor relationship. Many of these problems are not found in mentor relationships between men, because of the differences in socialization processes for the two sexes. Mentor relationships between men and women are less common, but problems exist in these relationships as well, as we have seen.

There can occur problems, however, which are not related to the sex of the individuals involved in the mentor relationship. These problems are related to the nature of the mentor relationship itself.

Vance alludes to the potential problems that may occur because of the parental nature of the mentor relationships.[22] The mentor in the "parent" role may be overprotective of the protégé (child). The protégé has to be assisted to achieve success and, ultimately, independence in his or her career. The mentor who is reluctant to encourage the protégé to take risks, such as presenting a paper at a national meeting, or writing a controversial article for publication, contributes to the dependence of the person being mentored.

The Jewel Companies executives described how their mentor relationships involved much give-and-take. In one instance, the protégé was allowed to make a rather serious mistake, since the mentor firmly believed that learning from one's own mistakes was an effective way of learning. Each of the executives, when in the role of protégé, was encouraged to take risks and to think for himself.

Overprotectiveness can take the form of shielding the protégé from persons who do not think or act in the same way as the mentor. The mentor may try to "protect" the protégé from hearing ideas that differ from the mentor's. The executives from Jewel described frequent discussions with their mentors about ideas and approaches that differed from those espoused by the mentor. The protégé was encouraged to challenge his mentor because the older person had enough self-confidence to be able to tolerate views that differed from his own. These protégés reported checking out ideas only when they thought it necessary, rather than at the behest of the mentor.

None of the respondents in either Vance's study or in the Roche study reported any overprotectiveness on the part of their mentors. However, in neither case were negative aspects of mentor relationships specifically studied.

Nonetheless, despite the difficulties that may occur in mentor relationships, the benefits of mentorship generally outweigh the problems. Both mentor and protégé must be aware of the problems that may arise in the relationship. Forewarned, then, both can act to minimize the damaging effects on the relationship.

SUMMARY

The mentor relationship is an idea whose time has come in the nursing profession. Mentorship can help develop tomorrow's nursing leaders. Protégés can assume responsibility for the future of the nursing profession more capably if they have learned the profession's values from individuals who have themselves been nursing leaders.

The profession will grow and mature if the wisdom of today's leaders is transmitted to the leaders of tomorrow. In addition to the intense personal satisfaction to be gained from women helping women and nurses helping nurses, mentor relationships are essential if the nursing profession is to progress in the future.

NOTES

1. Eliza G.C. Collins and Patricia Scott, "Everyone Who Makes It Has a Mentor," *Harvard Business Review* 56, no. 4 (July-August 1978): 89–101.

2. Gerard R. Roche, "Much Ado about Mentors," *Harvard Business Review* 57, no. 1 (January-February 1979): 14-28.

3. *Ibid.*, p. 15.

4. Collins and Scott, "Everyone Who Makes It Has a Mentor," p. 89.

5. Gail Sheehy, *Passages: Predictable Crises of Adult Life* (New York: Dutton, 1974), p. 189.

6. Margaret Hennig and Anne Jardim, *The Managerial Woman* (New York: Pocket Books, 1977), p. 27.

7. Lucie Young Kelly, *Dimensions of Professional Nursing*, 4th ed. (New York: Macmillan, 1981), p. 348.

8. Kathleen M. May, Afaf Ibrahim Meleis, and Patricia Winstead-Fry, "Mentorship for Scholarliness: Opportunities and Dilemmas," *Nursing Outlook*, January 1982, pp. 22-28.

9. *Ibid.*, p. 22.

10. Connie Vance, "A Group Profile of Contemporary Influentials in American Nursing," (Ed. D. Dissertation, Teachers College, Columbia University, 1977).

11. Patty Hawken, "Growing Our Own: A Way to Prepare Deans," *Nursing Outlook*, March 1980, p. 171.

12. Barbara Ann Larson, "An Exploratory Study of the Relationship of Job Satisfaction of Nursing Leaders in Hospital Settings Who Have Had a Mentor Relationship and Those Who Have Not," (Unpublished manuscript, Bellevue: University of Washington, 1980).

13. Roche, "Much Ado about Mentors," p. 24.

14. D. Levinson, *The Seasons of a Man's Life* (New York: Knopf, 1978), p. 98.

15. Connie N. Vance, "The Mentor Connection," *The Journal of Nursing Administration*, April 1982, pp. 7-13.

16. Roche, "Much Ado about Mentors," p. 20.
17. *Ibid.*, p. 28.
18. Vance, "The Mentor Connection," p. 10.
19. Hawken, "Growing Our Own," pp. 170-172.
20. Roche, "Much Ado about Mentors," p. 15.
21. Hennig and Jardim, *The Managerial Woman*, p. 33.
22. Vance, "The Mentor Connection," p. 8.

Chapter 5

Networking for Political Impact

Linda J. Shinn

There's no better place to practice your newly acquired or more finely tuned networking skills than in the political or legislative arena. For it is in this arena that people-to-people contacts or "who you know" can result in control over the expenditure of billions of governmental dollars; the election or defeat of candidates for political office; and the articulation of public policy in health, education, labor, and other arenas.

According to Davis et al., "At the federal level, about 2,500 health related bills and resolutions are introduced during every two year Congressional session. While only 2 percent of these are enacted into law, many have the potential to affect nursing."[1] In one midwestern state, in a two-year period, some 2,600 bills were introduced into the state legislature and approximately 10 percent had the potential to influence nurses and the practice of nursing. Clearly, then, developing and using one's contacts in the political arena can be not only beneficial but critical to the expansion of nursing's power and authority in society.

Politics can be defined as the mustering of monetary and human resources to influence the allocation of societal resources. The nursing community has fostered its participation in politics in two ways. First, since the early 1900s, the profession has lobbied legislative bodies to enact, amend, or repeal laws. Second, more recently, the profession has engaged in endorsing candidates for office in an effort to influence election outcomes.

United States Senator Daniel Inouye notes in his foreword to the book *Politics in Nursing* that "Politics in a real sense is the people who take the time to participate."[2] This chapter, then, focuses on the cultivation of networking skills to help nurses, in greater numbers, become the people who participate in making decisions about the allocation of societal resources.

DETERMINING THE NEED FOR POLITICAL INVOLVEMENT

"Many nurses consider political action to be unprofessional, unwomanly and unnecessary."[3] However, the need for involvement by nurses in the political or legislative arena can best be demonstrated by a brief review of several significant historical events in the past 80-plus years.

Early in the twentieth century, the issue of a standardized educational and regulatory system for nurses necessitated the organization of state nurses' associations to work for passage of nurse practice acts. No nurse would enjoy the benefits of licensure today had it not been for the political action of nurses in the early 1900s.

A modern-day example of the need for involving oneself in politics occurred during the administration of President Gerald Ford. Ford twice vetoed legislation that provided federal funding for nursing education in the United States. On both occasions, nurses recognized that the absence of federal funding to prepare nurses would ultimately jeopardize the health care of the public, as fewer nurses would be available to practice in hospitals, nursing homes, and other health care settings. Further, graduate programs to prepare nurses for careers in administration, education, and research would be seriously hampered without financial help from the federal government.

On both occasions, state nurses' associations were contacted by the American Nurses' Association's (ANA) Washington office to enlist the support of nurses and interested others to call, write, or visit members of the U.S. Congress urging them to override the vetoes. The state nurses' associations rallied to the challenge by contacting schools of nursing, nurse employers, specialty nursing organizations, news media, and individual nurses to assist in the effort. Congressional offices reported voluminous contacts by nurses.[4] Through the leadership of the ANA and its network of state nurses' associations, the vetoes were overridden by the Congress.

More recently, the licensure of nurses has been threatened as state boards of nursing are evaluated by state legislatures to determine whether or not the boards should continue to exist. This evaluation process has been dubbed "sunset" evaluation or review. Sunset evaluation has become a tool for state legislatures to use in determining whether or not agencies of state government are fulfilling the purposes for which they were established, with an aim toward decreasing the size of government and its cost. State agencies, such as boards of nursing, are being reviewed to determine whether or not they are protecting the public through the licensure process or, as some have suggested, protecting the professions by regulating entry and restricting competition in the marketplace by limited definitions of practice.

In some states, sunset evaluation is merely a review of agency activities. In other states, sunset inspection can result in the termination or restructuring of agencies. The spectre of termination or restructuring of boards of nursing has generated a great deal of concern in the nursing community.

The termination of a state board of nursing may mean the loss of mobility for nurses as endorsement of licenses from state to state could be curtailed. Further, licensure of new graduates could be halted and, in instances where reimbursement for services depends upon licensure, such reimbursement may cease. Moreover, the public would no longer be assured that the nurses caring for them were even minimally competent to practice. Schools of nursing would be required neither to have uniform curricula nor to meet minimum standards to operate.

Attempts at restructuring boards of nursing during sunset review could prove as deadly as the termination option. The near loss of the New Hampshire Board of Nursing is a good example. Legislators in New Hampshire received a report from their legislative staff recommending the termination of the Board of Nursing. In the next legislative session the New Hampshire legislature failed to reauthorize the Board of Nursing and it was scheduled to be disbanded on March 31, 1982.

Subsequently, the New Hampshire Nurses' Association, in coalition with other nursing organizations and other groups of nurses from around the country, convinced the New Hampshire Governor to call a special session of the New Hampshire legislature, in part, to authorize the continuation of the Board of Nursing. The Board of Nursing was ultimately reauthorized by the New Hampshire legislature.[5] Threats to nurse licensure, nursing practice, and nursing education will increase as competition for societal resources becomes keener. Such threats vividly demonstrate that the very existence of the profession of nursing and the welfare of its members depend heavily on the political involvement of nurses.

DECIDING THE EXTENT OF POLITICAL INVOLVEMENT

Nurses are among the more active segments of the United States citizenry in voting. A Nurses' Coalition for Action in Politics (N-CAP) survey reveals that 91 percent of the registered nurse population surveyed is registered to vote, compared with 70 percent of the adult population generally.[6] Recent statistics reveal that 1 in 44 registered women voters is a registered nurse.[7] Obviously, nurses are interested in participating in the selection of persons who represent them at various levels of government.

What is needed in the nursing profession, however, is a greater number of nurses willing to seek public office and the influence attendant to such officeholders. Billions of dollars are spent each year at all levels of government for health care and health manpower. Competition for health care dollars is becoming keener. The people who have control of these scarce dollars will shape health policy. The influence of nursing in the health care system will be enhanced only when nursing has a greater say on how and where health care dollars are spent. Holding public office is one of the best ways to mold health policy and the subsequent expenditure of monies. At present, according to Kalisch and Kalisch, approximately 10 percent of all elective offices in the United States are held by women.[8] Approximately 31 nurses nationwide hold some type of elected office.[9]

Depending upon where you are in fulfilling your personal and professional goals, voting may be the extent of your current political involvement. However, short of running for office, you may be able to become more politically involved than you think. For instance, if you know the positions on health/nursing issues of the candidates you plan to vote for, you can influence the vote of colleagues, family, or friends. For example, the following conversation might take place between you and a colleague during a coffee break:

> *You:* I had a fantastic experience over the weekend. I spent about 15 minutes with Representative Ritter. I'm going to support his candidacy for reelection and I hope you will, too.
>
> *Colleague:* You know he's running against Representative Pen in the primary. Both of them have been quite supportive of nursing during their years in office. I sure wish the Congressional redistricting had not resulted in pitting them against each other.
>
> *You:* Me, too, but Ritter is in the best position to be of the greatest help to nursing. He chairs the House Public Health Committee and that's where most of the legislation we are interested in is assigned for hearing. Also, he has consistently championed amendments to the Nurse Practice Act that give us more autonomy in nursing practice and less overall control of our practice by physicians. The other thing I like about him is his willingness to listen to nursing's viewpoints about issues. He will change his mind about things if he gets good input and convincing data.
>
> *Colleague:* The key in what you've said is Ritter's position as Chairman of the House Public Health Committee. Pen does not hold any health-related committee assignments. You're right, retaining Ritter in the House is important to nursing.

You also can give money, a few dollars or many, to the candidate or political party of your choice or write a letter to a legislator on an issue of interest to you.

Perhaps a moderate amount of political involvement suits your needs at the moment. Modest political activity might include:

- volunteering to work at political party headquarters
- volunteering time to work in the campaign of a preferred candidate for office
- participating in a political party convention as a delegate
- attending precinct meetings to get to know the local "politicos" in your area
- attending a hearing held by your state or local government on an issue of interest to you

Headquarters Work

Volunteer work at a political party headquarters might include answering the telephone, opening the mail, stuffing envelopes, or licking stamps. Such work gives the volunteer the opportunity to meet and make contacts with other volunteers, party officials, and officeholders. Keep in mind that work at party headquarters has peaks and valleys. The amount of work to be done increases as election time or party convention time nears.

Campaign Work

Volunteering to work in a candidate's campaign has several advantages. First, you will meet a lot of people who will be useful to involve in your political network. Such people might include political party chairpersons, media reporters, pollsters, and fund raisers. Second, you'll have a firsthand opportunity to learn the details of conducting a campaign, which can be put to good use if you run for office at some future time. Campaign work also gives you the opportunity to influence or shape your candidate's views about health-related matters. You might even be asked to help in drafting a candidate's position statement on health issues. To volunteer to work in a candidate's campaign is as easy as telephoning the candidate's campaign headquarters, identifying yourself, and offering your time.

One registered nurse reports that she attended a luncheon where a candidate for Congress spoke. At the conclusion of the luncheon, the nurse introduced herself to the candidate and offered to work in his upcoming election campaign. The offer was accepted on the spot.

Another nurse reports sitting next to her Congressman on an airplane. She took the opportunity to volunteer to work in his reelection campaign and to enlist some of her colleagues to do the same. Again, the offer was accepted.

Convention Participation

Usually, participating in a political party convention as a delegate requires being elected. Although delegate selection may vary from state to state or community to community, the process in your locale can quickly be identified by telephoning local party officials, the local League of Women Voters, the local library, or the local election board.

If you are not elected as a delegate on your first try, don't give up. Keep trying and as you develop recognition and a network in the political party you probably will win that delegate seat.

There are at least three reasons for being a full participant in a political party convention. First, you will have a say in slating candidates to run for office. This is a good place to influence the selection of a nurse. Second, you will have a voice in developing the party platform or positions on a variety of political, social, and health-related issues. Third, you will have an excellent opportunity to expand your political network by meeting both party leaders and party followers.

Precinct Meetings

In order to attend a political party precinct meeting, you need to identify the precinct you vote in. Generally, your precinct number will appear on your voter registration card. Precinct meetings usually focus on discussion of the candidates for office in a particular area and getting to know them, how to get out the vote on election day, and selecting the appropriate persons to head county and state political party offices. Precinct officers can expect a great deal of lobbying urging them to support specific candidates for political party office. Individuals active in precinct work can anticipate doing door-to-door solicitation for party nominees, driving in car pools or running child care services on election day, telephoning party supporters to get out the vote, and distributing campaign literature at polling places.

One community health nurse reports that she sought out a precinct official at her assigned voting place. While a precinct official for her political party was not present, an official for the opposing party was on hand. This official introduced her to other precinct officials and scores of officeholders and party workers. Subsequently, the nurse met the precinct committeeman for her own party, attended precinct functions, and eventually became vice-chairperson of her precinct.

Hearings

Government at all levels has become increasingly accessible to the general public. Many actions taken by government require public input at some stage. For example, state legislatures usually conduct public hearings on proposed legislation as a first step in the legislative process. Agencies in the executive branch of government, such as state boards of nursing, are customarily required to conduct public hearings on proposed rules or regulations. Attending a public hearing can provide you with opportunities to gather information, to speak for or against an issue, and to meet people who shape public policy, thus expanding your political network.

Information about hearings on matters before the legislative or executive branch of government can be obtained in a variety of ways. Most newspapers carry a public notice column that may include public hearing announcements. Also, newspapers frequently carry detailed information about matters under consideration by city, town, or county government. Newspapers published in the capital city of most states are excellent sources of information about state government activities. Although you may not live in the capital city of your state, your local library will undoubtedly subscribe to the newspaper(s) published in the capital city.

Don't overlook your state or district nurses' association or state board of nursing as a source of information about public hearings on matters related to nursing. The names and addresses of state nurses' associations and boards of nursing are listed in the directory issue of the *American Journal of Nursing,* published yearly in April.

Giving Testimony

If you give testimony at a public hearing these guidelines should be followed:

- Know your audience
- Know your subject matter
- Address only one subject at a time
- Do not become argumentative

- Do not read your testimony
- Prepare copies of your remarks to distribute

Know Your Audience

Getting to know the audience you plan to testify before is easy. If you are to give testimony to members of a committee of the state legislature, attend one or two committee meetings prior to the time you will appear before the committee. This activity will give you the opportunity to become familiar with the committee members by name and face. You also will have the opportunity to see how the committee operates. Note modes of operation for committee procedures. Does the committee require those who give testimony to sign up in advance of the committee meeting? Do persons appearing before the committee sit in a special place in the hearing room? Do committee members make use of written statements presented to them or do they toss them aside? Does the committee chair impose a time limit on presenters? Are witnesses questioned by committee members? Can witnesses offer additional comments after their testimony has been given?

Obtain background information on committee members. Frequently, biographical sketches of legislators at the state or federal level will be available through state Chambers of Commerce, statehouse information bureaus, legislators' offices, or from political party headquarters. Don't forget the members of your network—and your mentor. Background information can give you a clue as to the type of questions the audience might ask. For example, a legislator serving on a hospital board of trustees will have information and insights that may prompt him or her to ask a nurse testifier more detailed and technical questions about a health care issue than a legislator who has no health background.

Know the Subject Matter

Familiarity with the subject matter you testify about is crucial. If you are well versed about the subject being addressed you will be at ease in presenting your case, articulate in responding to questions, and convincing in presenting arguments for or against the issue. A good grasp of the matter at hand will also establish you as a resource person to be turned to at a future time.

When you know the ins and outs of the issue you are addressing you are less likely to make errors in presenting facts or data. *Facts must be accurate.* Have citations for facts at hand. The spreading of erroneous information can jeopardize your cause as well as your credibility.

Clarity and brevity are good companions for the testifier. Often, the attention span of the audience will be limited. If your testimony comes to the point and contains understandable language, those listening to you will truly hear what you have to say. If you want to illustrate a point you are making, consider using an example known to your audience. Avoid technical terms with which listeners may not be familiar or that have to be defined in great detail.

Address One Subject

Generally, testimony should focus on a single subject. Zeroing in on a specific subject assists the presenter in being brief, clear, and concise. Covering too much ground in a presentation may result in losing the audience, rambling, or repetition.

Avoid Argument

Although you may know more about the subject than anyone else in the room, avoid the appearance of having a closed mind on the issue and avoid becoming argumentative. Demonstrating a willingness to listen to and to consider other points of view will leave a favorable impression on the audience. Becoming argumentative while testifying or responding to questions in an angry manner sets the stage for an unfavorable reaction and response to the presentation you make.

Learn to be persistent and firm in a pleasant manner. Often a dash of humor in a tense or emotion-laden situation will result in those you are speaking to not only hearing what you have to say but remembering you and what you said long after the hearing is over.

Do Not Read Your Testimony

Reading from a prepared statement does not enhance public testimony. The audience may get the impression that the presenter is reading someone else's words or, worse yet, giving another's point of view. On the other hand, memorized testimony may sound like a recording. While it may be desirable to have your remarks in writing, familiarity with the subject matter will help in presenting views in a self-assured, personal manner. Occasional referral to written remarks, if done in an unobtrusive manner, is appropriate and may be helpful in preserving the accuracy of facts and figures.

Prepare Copies of Remarks

Presenters of testimony differ in their opinions as to whether or not written testimony should be presented to an audience prior to the giving of the testimony or at the conclusion of the remarks. Persons who support the distribution of testimony in advance assert that having a document in hand aids the listener in following and comprehending the presentation being given. Those who oppose advance distribution of testimony state that the audience is too busy reading ahead or being distracted by the appearance of the written material to pay attention to what is being said.

The prudent testifier will decide upon the timing for distributing written remarks based upon the advance knowledge gathered about the habits of the audience. Also, the presenter may wish to distribute only an outline or highlights of the remarks made in order to focus the audience's attention upon the key points or arguments.

Many state nurses' associations sponsor "nurses' day" at the state legislature. Such events are excellent opportunities to become initiated to the workings of government and to attend or testify at a public hearing. On occasion, nursing organizations need to amass large numbers of nurses at the seat of state government to support or oppose an issue. Call your state nurses' association and let them know if you are willing to be "on call" to attend a public hearing.

RUNNING FOR PUBLIC OFFICE

If your goals and time permit, your political involvement might include holding public office. An accurate assessment of where your interests lie and the time you have available for pursuit of office can result in the height of political involvement, an elected or appointed office. Whether you seek office on the school board, hospital board, or in city, state, or federal government, the Nurses' Coalition for Action in Politics (N-CAP), the political action arm of the American Nurses' Association, recommends several guidelines:

- know all about the job you seek
- know all about the current officeholder's positions, decisions and supporting networks
- know the issues
- check the statistics from several recent elections and ask yourself: Is now the time to run? Is there a voting pattern in previous elections for or against the incumbent? Has the incumbent received a large majority of the votes cast in the past?
- know if the contest is partisan and how you get the party's nomination
- know federal, state or local election laws

- find out how much money was spent on previous elections
- make a list of contacts to call upon for aid. Do you know someone with campaign experience that you can call upon for help?
- cultivate the media in your area to get your name before the public
- contact the political action arm for nurses in your state for help[10]

Knowing the Job

Information you will want to know about the job you are seeking includes the following: How much time will it take to fulfill the responsibilities of the office? Is there a per diem allowance for holding the office? How much of your own money will you need to spend in fulfilling the responsibilities of the job? Are clerical services or support staff services provided? Is extensive travel required? What is the term of office? Who are you responsible to and what are the procedures for getting the job done?

One registered nurse prepared several years in advance to run for the state legislature. She worked as a lobbyist for the League of Women Voters and on the staff of the state legislature to gain knowledge about the job she sought.

Knowing the Officeholder

You'll want to gather data about how long the current officeholder has been in office, whether or not the person has been reelected by wide vote margins, if there was viable opposition in previous primary and general elections, if the individual consistently has been slated to run for office by his or her political party or if he or she has been bypassed by the slating process or been defeated by other party nominees in the slating process, and what his or her voting record has been on issues of major importance to constituents. Such issues might include property taxes, equal rights for women, busing, abortion, and so forth.

Resources for doing your homework on the current officeholder include newspapers, journals or minutes that cover the proceedings of the body in which the officeholder serves, previous campaign literature of the officeholder, interviews with party officials or persons who have previously sought or held the office. Also, you may find it helpful to talk to several constituents of the present officeholder to determine how satisfied they are with the job being done.

Knowing the Issues

Issues before the body you wish to serve in can be readily identified by attending meetings of the body; by reading newspapers, meeting minutes, or journals prepared by the body; by listening to TV or radio news; and by talking to others holding the office you aspire to. For example, you may plan to run for school board. By attending meetings of the school board in your community, the parent-teacher organization at your children's school, and reading the newspapers published in your area, you will probably discover, as one nurse candidate for school board did, that most of the school board's work revolves around money: money for teacher salaries, money for school building maintenance, money for textbooks, and money for busing children to school. The nurse candidate for school board had been politically active in her community for a number of years and had developed a great deal of knowledge about school funding. She was well prepared to seek and win a seat on the local school board.

Checking Previous Election Data

Local election boards, political party offices, or newspapers are good sources of statistics about previous elections. The statistics will reveal whether or not the voters in your area repeatedly favor one political party over another. If the voting pattern in your community is consistently Republican and you want to run for office on the Democratic ticket you know you may have an uphill battle and a slim chance of winning.

Previous election data may reveal that the incumbent is winning reelection by a smaller and smaller margin every time he or she runs for office. Such a trend may be a signal that the time is right, or may soon be right, for the incumbent to be defeated. On occasion, officeholders will not seek reelection. This, too, can be a signal that now is the time to run. You will want to be sensitive to the fact that there may be an "heir apparent" to the job being vacated by an incumbent. The political party network of the incumbent in your community is the best source of this information.

Understanding the Contest

Information gleaned about previous elections and the political habits of your community are your best clues as to whether or not the office you're interested in being elected to is fraught with political party considerations. For example, obtaining the party's nomination may be as simple as asking for it or as complex as competing against a myriad of others wanting to run for the same spot. In some locales, political parties hold slating conventions where persons must be nominated and voted upon in order to be slated as a candidate to run for office.

One of the best ways to get your party's nomination is to prove yourself a loyal party supporter. To accomplish this, you must be a worker in party affairs, such as the election campaigns of others and voter registration drives, and knowledgeable about and an ardent supporter of the party's platform. Political activities at the local level are key to building a network of personal and professional influence. It is at the local level that you will meet the people who can make things happen for you and propel you into office.

Knowing the Laws

Information about the election laws in your area can be obtained from political party headquarters or officials, election boards, or libraries. Also, the secretary of state or attorney general in many states have responsibility for overseeing state election laws and are, therefore, good sources of information about these laws. Information about federal election laws can be obtained through your U.S. representative, the Federal Election Commission, or the local library.

Election laws detail such things as requirements for having your name placed on the ballot, deadlines that must be met in filing your candidacy for office, and campaign spending limitations and reporting requirements related to campaign contributions. Election laws also may describe the parameters for conducting primary and general elections, contesting election outcomes, and determining legislative districts and voter registration.

Getting Money To Finance a Campaign

One of the most crucial aspects of running for office is having enough money to wage a successful campaign. The amount of money you spend on a campaign will depend on the office you are running for, the competition, the size of the constituency to be influenced, election laws, and the campaign coffers of your political party.

If you are running for school board, you may find that bumper stickers, election posters, and leaflets are enough. If you are running for state treasurer, you will probably find it necessary to advertise in the media. Obviously, the size of your constituency, when running for a state office as opposed to a local office, will necessitate a greater outlay of money, as you will be trying to influence the votes of a larger number of people.

Money for campaigns can be raised in a variety of ways. Fund raisers include such things as cocktail parties, dinners, car washes, or raffles.

Individual or group contributions are also sources of funds. Any candidate for office should check applicable federal, state, or local laws to determine whether or not there are restrictions on the methods for raising funds and how funds raised are to be accounted for and reported.

Listing Your Contacts

Your business card collection or notebook that details those in your professional and personal network is a good place to start for making a list of contacts to call upon to help you in your campaign for office. Also, your family and neighbors might be a good source to turn to for help. More than likely, persons active in your political party can be called upon for aid. Political party workers or officials usually will have valuable campaign experience that you can tap. Call your state or district nurses' association and ask for the names, addresses, and telephone numbers of other nurses who have run for or held offices in your state.

Frequently, women's groups in your community will sponsor seminars on running for office. Contact local chapters of the National Organization for Women, Women in Communications, or Republican or Democratic women's groups for additional information.

Cultivating the Media

Cultivating the media may take the form of appearing on television or radio or being interviewed by local papers. Letters to the editors of local newspapers or magazines about issues of interest to you or your community are also routes to gaining public name recognition.

There are a number of ways to gain radio or TV coverage. For example, you may be active in a local chapter of the American Heart Association and have the opportunity to appear on a radio call-in show to answer questions about heart disease or hypertension. You might seek the chance to reply in person to a TV or radio editorial that you did not agree with or want to lend support to. Your community activities may include work for the local humane society, which entails participating in a telethon to raise money for the society.

If you want to run for office, don't pass up such opportunities for media exposure. Keep in mind, too, that the television media will portray every nuance about your person. Thus, it is a good idea to be well groomed. Do not wear white when having your picture taken or appearing on television. A dark color is much more effective. A two-piece business suit in a conservative color with appropriate accessories is your best bet for a television appearance. Neatly groomed hair is essential. There is nothing more distracting to a television audience than an individual constantly fidgeting with his or her hair.

Getting Help

At present, 36 states have groups of nurses who have formed political action committees (PACs) to help people get elected to office and to support the reelection of incumbents supportive to nursing.[11] The nurses' political action organization in your state may contribute money to your campaign or manpower to help hand out campaign literature, staff a telephone bank, or provide expertise on how to run a campaign. The nurses' association in your state can put you in touch with the state PAC.

If you are organized, and plan your time wisely, you can be politically involved. The choice about the extent is up to you—a little or a lot!

IDENTIFYING POLITICIANS YOU NEED TO KNOW

After you have determined the extent of your political involvement, you will want to identify those politicians who will facilitate your political commitments. If the extent of your involvement is voting, you'll want to familiarize yourself with candidates for office and their viewpoints. Some resources for this undertaking are local newspapers, media events such as televised candidate debates or radio call-in shows, "Meet the Candidate" nights at local shopping centers, fish fries or neighborhood coffees, or door-to-door campaigns.

If your political involvement includes letter writing about a piece of legislation before the U.S. Congress, you will want to know the identity of your U.S. senator and representative. If you want to influence the actions taken by the state legislature, you will need to know the identity of your state representatives, members of the assembly, or senators. This information is available through community newspapers, local libraries, the local League of Women Voters, Chamber of Commerce, or political party headquarters. You may wish to use one of your established networks with a colleague or neighbor to determine this information.

The identity of state legislators and members of the U.S. House of Representatives can be obtained with greater ease if you know the number(s) of your legislative district(s). The number of your district represented in the state assembly may differ from the number of the district your state senator represents. Frequently, Congressional districts are numbered differently from state legislative districts. U.S. senators do not represent particular districts.

If you do not have the number of your legislative district, ask for it when you obtain the names of your elected state and federal officials. An inquiry as to the identity of your state representative or assembly member might go like this:

> *You:* Good morning, I'm Elizabeth Frank and I'm calling to find out who my state representative is. I live in House District 46.
>
> *Political Party Headquarters (PPH):* Thank you. I'll check. Your district is represented by three people, Representative Jon Fritz, Representative Frank Dovis, and Representative Florence Carrier.

If you do not know the number of your House district, you may have to supply your address and the name of the township in which you live. When obtaining the names of those who represent you be sure to get their addresses to have on hand for future contacts.

Perhaps you are interested in a noise abatement ordinance under consideration by the city council or town board in the city or town where you live. Information about the identity of the council or board members, sponsors of the ordinance, who you should write to in support of or in opposition to the ordinance, or when and where a public meeting will be held on the proposed ordinance can be obtained by telephoning the mayor's or town manager's office.

If you plan to be active in politics to the extent of running for office or participating in a political campaign, you will want to know local political party officials, including precinct committee members or ward chairpersons. Often these officials have a great deal of influence over who is nominated to run for office or who will serve as political party convention delegates. Getting to know local party officials can only strengthen and enhance your network. The identity of such officials can be obtained by contacting the local Democratic or Republican headquarters. Contacts already established in your neighborhood or at work also might be tapped for this information.

Identifying politicians important to your political network is easy. All you need is a telephone and telephone book. Once you have the information about who these officials are and who should be contacted to influence specific issues, keep the information updated and handy. The notebook or file box you're using to keep information on the people in your network (see Chapter 2) is perfect for keeping data on politicians. Organizing the information by topic should be the most helpful. For example, the following topic headings might be used:

- city or town officials
- state officials
- national officials

The notes under the topic heading "state officials" might look like those displayed on the note card in Exhibit 5-1.

Your system, whatever it is, should be organized to be of the most help to you. The system should be kept updated as your elected officials change and as your interests and priorities change.

ESTABLISHING AND MAINTAINING RELATIONSHIPS

Once you've identified the politicians who belong in your network, it's time to get ready to meet them. There are several steps to follow in meeting a politician. They are:

- prepare for the meeting
- meet the individual
- establish rapport
- obtain information
- provide information
- summarize and close the meeting
- evaluate the meeting

Preparing for the Meeting

It is helpful to have background information on the politicians you want to meet. For example, what are their occupations? What community organ-

---

Exhibit 5–1 Organizing Information

State Official	
Jon Fritz	Political Party: Democratic
1414 Guilford	Office: Member, House of
Rex, Indiana 46014	Representatives; Majority
Office Phone: (317) 666-2134	Leader
	Occupation: Retired

Other: Active in senior citizen organizations. Wife is a nurse.
Authored amendments to Nurse Practice Act in 1981 to add consumer to Board of Nursing.

izations are they involved in? What political party are they members of? Do they have spouses or other relatives who are nurses?

If the politician you want to meet is a legislator, the following information would be helpful: How long has he or she served in the legislature, assembly, or Congress? What committee assignments does the legislator have? Has the legislator introduced or sponsored legislation related to nursing or health care?

Personal information, such as church membership, might help you find common ground for meeting a politician or for establishing rapport. Information about longevity as a legislator will give you some idea as to the status, power, or influence the legislator may have with his or her legislative colleagues. If the legislator you want to meet has an interest in health care or nursing, you will have additional common ground for exchange of information and ideas. Knowing whether or not the politician you want to meet has a nurse relative will give you a clue as to how you should approach him or her. It also lets you know that your views or ideas may be validated or discussed with the nurse relative, who might or might not be supportive.

Be sure to know what you want to gain from meeting a politician. Do you want to become more involved in a political party by volunteering to work in a political campaign? Do you want to influence a piece of legislation or government regulations? Do you want the politician to speak at the next chapter meeting of Sigma Theta Tau?

If you want to volunteer to work in a campaign be sure you know how much time you have to give to the effort. Also, take your business cards to the meeting so that you might leave a ready reference for future contacts. A meeting related to influencing legislation necessitates familiarity with the matters to be discussed. Know the bill number and the status of the bill at the moment. Is the legislator you plan to meet in a position to do your bidding? What expenditures are involved? If you plan to ask a politician to speak at a meeting of your Sigma Theta Tau Chapter, know what issues you want the politician to address, as well as the date, time, and place of the meeting.

Meeting the Politician

Armed with information about the politician you want to meet and the purpose for such a meeting, you are ready to go. Face-to-face contact is always best for a first meeting. A face-to-face meeting gives you the opportunity to size up the politician, to get immediate verbal and nonverbal feedback on the issues discussed, and to gain recognition in the eyes of the politician so that you might start becoming a part of his or her network.

The first meeting should focus on getting to know each other. The meeting might take place at lunch, a neighborhood social, or the politician's office. If you want to get acquainted with your state senator or representative, invite him or her to your home for coffee and invite your neighbors or nurse colleagues who are also constituents of the legislator to the coffee. A person in your network may already know the politician you want to meet and be willing to introduce you. Another way to meet an officeholder is to telephone his or her office and set up an appointment.

An appointment phone call might go like this:

You: Hello, this is Mickey Francis. I'm calling to make an appointment with Senator Woods. July 19 is the date most convenient for me.

Appointment Clerk (AC): Senator Woods can see you at 2 P.M. on the 19th. Is that convenient for you?

You: Yes, thank you.

A.C.: May I ask what you would like to see the Senator about?

You: Yes. I'd like to speak with him about the recodification of Michigan's Public Health Laws. I'm a registered nurse and quite interested in the proposed revisions to the laws and how the changes will influence the Nurse Practice Act.

A.C.: Fine.

You: Thank you for your help. I'll look forward to meeting Senator Woods in the state office building at 2 P.M. on July 19. Goodbye.

If meeting the politician for the first time takes place over the telephone, be sure to identify yourself and the purpose of your call. Come to the point at once. If a lengthy conversation is necessary, make an appointment to meet the person telephoned to continue the discussion. It's good to keep in mind that a politician's time is as precious as yours.

Establishing Rapport

The establishment of rapport with another individual, including a politician, takes time and effort. If you are articulate about your concerns, honest, and willing to listen to opposing views, you will have little trouble establishing a harmonious relationship. The development of such a relationship takes time and won't necessarily be accomplished in one meeting. On occasion, the chemistry between a nurse and a politician may negate the creation of rapport. If this happens to you, recognize it for what it is and determine whether or not future contacts would be worthwhile. It may be that one of your colleagues could build a better association with this politician.

Obtaining and Giving Information

Once you have met the politicians of your choice, keep in contact with them. Exchange business cards at your first meeting so you can readily be in touch in the future. You may be contacting these individuals to obtain information or to give information. Be sure the information you provide is accurate and up to date. Establish credibility and visibility and you'll be contacted again and again by politicians who need information about nursing or the subject matter in which you have expertise.

Davis et al. suggest that a neat, factual briefing sheet of one to two pages should be prepared to leave with the politician. The sheet should detail succinctly the facts or concerns you have about the issue being addressed.[12] If you are asked for information you do not have, offer to get it, and specify a time at which the additional information will be provided. See Exhibit 5-2 for an example.

If you are meeting a politician to obtain information, it is usually good practice to ask for the information "up front." For example, if you want to know how a legislator plans to vote on a particular issue, ask. Generally, "beating around the bush" or engaging in "charades" to get information results in obtaining misinformation or no information at all, not to mention alienating the individual and jeopardizing your credibility for the future.

It is a good practice to listen for other information that might be transmitted in addition to the knowledge you've set out to gather. Recently, one nurse telephoned a legislator to ask for his position on a bill to change certain conditions for registered nurse license renewal. While the legislator promised to consider the issue and did not have a firm position at the time of the call, he advised the nurse that he did not support the licensure of health care providers generally and that he would discuss the merits of the proposed legislation with a physician member of the legislature. Certainly, this additional information was helpful to the nurse in preparing for future contacts with this particular legislator. It also is the kind of information that should be given to state nurses' association lobbyists and political action arms of state nurses' associations.

Closing the Meeting

A good habit to develop in concluding a substantive meeting with an officeholder is to summarize the information you have received or given.

Exhibit 5–2 Additional Information

1222 North Heather
Indianapolis, Indiana 46224
February 16, 1981

The Honorable John Brown
Indiana Senate
Senate Post Office
State House
Indianapolis, Indiana 46204

Dear Senator Brown:

At your request I have gathered information related to the nurse's duty to report changes in patient conditions. As you know, the law controlling the practice of nursing in the State is the Indiana State Board of Nurses' Registration and Nursing Education Act. The definitions of registered nurse and licensed practical nurse and their practices are found in the act.

George D. Pozgar's text, *Legal Aspects of Health Care Administration,* published in 1979 by Aspen Systems Corporation, cites several cases dealing with patient condition reporting. One of the cases cited is Citizens' Hospital Association v. Schoulin, 48 Ala. 101, 262 So. 2d 303 (1972). In this case, the court held "that the evidence was sufficient to sustain a jury verdict that the hospital's nurse was negligent in failing to apprise the doctor of all the patient's symptoms, in failing to conduct a proper examination of the plaintiff and in failing to follow the directions of a physician." Another case is Goff v. Doctor's General Hospital, 166 Cal. App. 2d 314, P. 2d 29 (1958), in which the court held "that nurses who knew that a woman they were attending was bleeding excessively were negligent in failing to report the circumstances so prompt and adequate measures could be taken to safeguard her life."

I have also enclosed for your information, *Standards for Medical–Surgical Nursing Practice* and the *Code for Nurses* published by the American Nurses' Association. If I can be of further help, please call me.

Sincerely,

Linda J. Shinn

Linda J. Shinn, R.N.

Enc: (2)

If you have been promised an action, confirm it at the meeting's close. If you have promised to take an action, reiterate your intent to do so. Specify a time at which you plan to follow up on your meeting. For example, you might say: "I'll obtain the numbers of registered nurses in Henson County and deliver the numbers to your office on Friday." Or "I appreciate your willingness to vote for the school enterers immunization legislation."

A lull in the conversation or searching for something else to say are good indicators that it is time to conclude the meeting. If you are in control of the meeting, bring it to a close. On occasion, the politician will take control of a meeting and bring it to a close by staging an interruption by a staff member or rising from a chair and changing the subject. Again, summarize the information you have received or given and reconfirm an action promised or one that you plan to take. Thank the politician for his or her time and depart. If another meeting seems indicated, ask to see the person responsible for appointment scheduling and arrange for another meeting time.

Evaluating the Meeting

After a meeting with a politician take a few moments to evaluate it. Did you accomplish what you set out to? Is there something you would do differently the next time? Is follow-up required? If so, when? Did you gain information that should be given to another individual in your network or your state nurses' association? Take a moment to make a few anecdotal notes in your "political" notebook or file box (see Exhibit 5-3).

A substantive meeting with your senator might evolve as follows:

You: Senator Snow, it's nice to see you again. I'm here today to urge you not to decrease funding for the colleges and universities in our state, particularly the schools of nursing.

Senator Snow: I'm receiving a great deal of pressure to support budget cuts in the interest of holding down our state's budgetary deficit and one of the places we plan to trim is in our state supported institutions' budgets.

You: Centralia University School of Nursing plans to offer a new master's program next fall in gerontological nursing. A cut in their budget at this time will seriously jeopardize starting the program.

Senator Snow: We're going to have to tighten our belts somehow. The state's financial future appears pretty bleak.

You: You've long championed the cause of quality nursing homes in our state and have publicly urged nurses and nursing

Exhibit 5–3 Anecdotal Notes of Meeting with Politician

Accomplishments: Senator Snow will probably take another look at budgetary allocations for colleges and universities, particularly Centralia University. Senator Snow has been informed about the gerontological nursing program to be offered by the school of nursing at Centralia University.

Do differently next time: Nothing

Follow-up: Get detailed budgetary breakdown for school of nursing at Centralia and proposed costs of master's program in gerontological nursing. Take information to Snow's office by March 2.

Information to be given to others: Call state nurses' association and report conversation with Snow. Advise SNA Snow may be willing to rethink his stance on state budget cuts for universities.

Anecdotal notes: Snow's press assistant's sister is a nurse.

homes to work together to find ways to increase the numbers of nurses employed in extended care facilities. One of the major things that influences where nurses seek employment is their knowledge and ability. Working with the elderly requires an in-depth knowledge of the aging process, nutrition, family relationships, and so forth. An educational program with an emphasis on how to care for the elderly population will assist registered nurses in becoming more knowledgeable about and comfortable in working with the elderly. The gerontological nursing program at Centralia will have a clinical practicum in five area nursing homes. I can't help but think that the program will generate more nurses interested in working with the elderly in nursing homes.

Senator Snow: How many students will be admitted to the program in the fall?

You: 20.

Senator Snow: Well, your points are well taken. Maybe we should take a closer look at the Centralia budget. Can you get me a detailed breakdown on the school of nursing's budget as well as a breakdown on the costs of the new program—within a week?

You: I can get the additional information for you. I do have a fact sheet with me that highlights the budgets of the schools of nursing in our state generally. Centralia's School of Nursing budget is included. I'll leave this fact sheet with you and get the additional information for you within a week.

Senator Snow: Great.

You: I appreciate the time you have given me this morning to talk about the budget issue.

Senator Snow: Thank you for coming to see me.

Often, communicating with politicians takes the written form. A well-written, accurate communique will help in establishing and maintaining political relationships. Timely written communications will keep the politicians of choice in your network.

Whether communicating as an individual or as a member of a special interest group, the following points should be adhered to:

- Spell the name of the person you are addressing correctly.
- Use the proper salutation and closing (see Exhibit 5-4). The salutation sets the tone of your letter and subsequently prompts the receiver's attention, reaction, and response.
- Personalize all communications. Cite *your* reason for or against an issue. Use personal examples to illustrate points.
- Type your letter only if your handwriting is not legible.
- Identify yourself clearly in the communication and give your voting address. If you are writing or telegramming on behalf of an organization or group, identify the affiliation.
- Identify the issue you are corresponding about. If legislation is involved, be sure to cite the name and number of the legislation.
- Deal with only one subject per communique.
- Know the subject matter you're writing about.
- Be brief, concise, and accurate.
- Give facts and your reasons for supporting or opposing an issue.
- Avoid emotionalism and threats.

Two sample letters appear in Exhibits 5-5 and 5-6.

Whether communicating in person or via letter or telegram be sure to say thank you: for listening to your concerns, for additional information, for a favor or a vote. Keep in mind that networking with a politician only when you want a favor is bad business. Networking, as mentioned previously, is a two-way street.

Exhibit 5–4 Letters to Politicians

Acceptable Salutations:

The Honorable John Adams
Indiana Senate
Senate Post Office
State House
Indianapolis, Indiana 46204

Dear Senator Adams:

or

The Honorable Doris Tag
Indiana House of Representatives
House Post Office
State House
Indianapolis, Indiana 46204

Dear Mrs. Tag:

or

The Honorable Stuart Smith
U.S. Senate
200 Russell Senate Office Building
Washington, D.C. 20515

Dear Senator Smith:

Acceptable closing:

Sincerely,

Belinda E. Puetz

Belinda E. Puetz, Ph.D., R.N.

APPLYING NETWORKING SKILLS TO CONTACTS WITH POLITICIANS

When you call upon a politician for something or when you give a politician something, you are networking. It is possible to network with a politician as an individual or as a member of a group. Since most politicians are men, however, and, by and large, members of the "old boys' net-

Exhibit 5–5 Sample Letter

1222 North Heather
Indianapolis, Indiana 46224
June 3, 1980

The Honorable Dave Evans
Member of Congress
438 Cannon Office Building
Washington, D.C. 20515

Dear Representative Evans:

As one of your constituents I am delighted to know that you plan to conduct a public hearing on the nursing shortage in Congressional District 6 on June 7. Since I will be out of the state attending a meeting and unable to participate in the hearing, I am addressing my comments to you in writing. The environments within which registered nurses practice and the salaries registered nurses are paid are going to have to improve markedly to ensure retention of RNs in active practice. Several striking examples can be cited. Recently, it has come to my attention that RNs in a large metropolitan hospital in Indiana are used as cleaning personnel and secretaries, their nursing education and skills taking a back seat to floor mopping and completing charge slips. Certainly, this practice environment is not conducive to RN retention.

An example of the tremendous pay injustices in nursing can be cited by comparing RN starting salaries at a facility in northeastern Indiana with factory floor sweepers in the same locale. The RNs are paid $6.01 per hour and the floor sweepers are paid $9.00 an hour.

These two striking examples, in my view, demonstrate why nurses leave nursing for other professions or fail to return to practice after taking a leave from employment.

Your public support for better salaries and practice conditions would be helpful. You are to be commended for conducting a hearing on nursing manpower and calling the public's attention to a matter that may well influence the quality and quantity of nursing care delivered in our community.

Sincerely,

Linda J. Shinn

Linda J. Shinn, R.N.

work," you may find that dealing with politicians as part of a group using the "old girls' network" is best.

One of nursing's best "old girls' networks" exists through state nurses' associations. Members of the Arizona Nurses' Association created the Arizona Nursing Network in 1977 to disseminate information regarding nursing and health care in Arizona, to increase political awareness among

Exhibit 5–6 Sample Letter

March 5, 1979

The Honorable Lawrence M. Borst
Indiana Senate
State House
Indianapolis, IN 46204

Dear Senator Borst:

It is my understanding that S.B. 489 may be called down for a second reading yet this week. This bill includes a number of amendments to the Nurse Practice Act among which is an amendment which requires that individuals who practice nursing acts must be licensed (with certain exceptions). I am in support of the bill because I believe it will help in ensuring that nursing services delivered in Indiana will be improved in quality. Under the current law individuals may practice nursing acts without a license. There are only 3 states and one territory remaining in the United States in which this situation is permitted to exist and Indiana is one of these. I have no statistics to offer you for consideration of the number of problems this situation has created. However, it is of concern to me that in this state individuals are allowed to practice nursing *without* the patients being ensured that the individuals providing them nursing care have met minimum standards; i.e., passed the five State Board licensing examinations, which are necessary for licensure. There have been a number of concerns registered about this bill, but I believe that they are unfounded. Those concerns and my responses to those concerns are as follows:

1. Nurses will lose their licenses. Response: No nurse will lose his or her license under this bill.
2. Unlicensed persons who are practicing nursing will not have an opportunity to obtain a license. Response: Individuals will have an opportunity to sit for the State Board licensing examinations if they have met the stipulations set forth in the Nurse Practice Act and in the Indiana State Board of Nurses' Registration and Nursing Education Rules and Regulations (these rules and regulations are by no means unreasonable).
3. Technicians in nursing homes and extended care facilities who have passed a medication course will not be allowed to administer medications. Response: They will certainly be allowed to do this according to the exclusion clause found in Section 17, No. 5 (Page 10, Lines 24–29). According to this exclusion, they may practice certain activities listed in the definition (Page 2, Lines 4–26) under supervision, which would include administering oral medications.
4. Physicians will not be able to delegate certain activities to their employees. Response: Physicians would be able to delegate certain activities as stipulated in exclusion clauses 5 and 6 in Section 17 on Page 10.

Exhibit 5–6 continued

In conclusion, should S.B. 489 be called down for a second reading, I urge you to support the bill as it is *currently* written (2/23/79). If you have any questions about 264-4412 (Secretary- 264-4413). Thank you very much for your consideration of my request.

Sincerely,

Juanita Laidig

Juanita Laidig, R.N.
8421 Del Prado Court
Indianapolis, IN 46227

JL: llm

cc: Linda J. Shinn, Associate Executive Director, I.S.N.A.
   Shirley Ross, President, I.S.B.N.R.N.E.

Source: Juanita M. Laidig, personal letter. Reprinted with permission from the author.

Arizona nurses, and to encourage nurses to participate in the legislative process. The Arizona Nursing Network at its inception consisted of some 20 organizations and 4,000 nurses and utilized a telephone tree to transmit information and to call nurses to action. The Arizona network has succeeded in making Arizona's legislators aware of nursing's concerns about numerous health-related issues.[13]

In Indiana, during the Indiana General Assembly's sunset evaluation of licensing boards, the Committee on Legislation of the Indiana State Nurses' Association (ISNA) established an ISNA member/state legislator communications network. The objectives of the network were "(1) to involve the ISNA member more directly in the legislative process, (2) to develop an ongoing legislator-ISNA member/constituent relationship, and (3) to inform members of the Indiana General Assembly about issues of concern to and positions of the ISNA."[14]

Legislators serving on Indiana's Sunset Evaluation Committee were "assigned" to ISNA member/volunteers who were their constituents. These ISNA members contacted their assigned legislators before the legislative session during which the sunset review of licensing boards took place and kept in touch with their legislators during the legislative session. The network can be credited, in part, with increasing nursing's visibility during the 1981 session of the Indiana General Assembly and the subsequent enactment of a mandatory nurse practice act.

We have already noted the situation in New Hampshire. It was the New Hampshire Nurses' Association's "Coalition of Action for Nursing" that influenced the New Hampshire Legislature to enact legislation to retain the New Hampshire Board of Nursing. The Coalition accomplished what it set out to do and its success can be attributed to creating a nursing network as follows:

> Their first task was to build a mailing list of every nurse in the state so they could spread their message. Then, they organized by county, naming organizational leaders to be responsible for nurses in the county contacting house and senate members about the measure. Through mailings, they provided lobbying information to each nurse and tips about how to call and approach the issue, with a feedback mechanism provided so that a central tally could be maintained. They also found legislators from both parties who were willing to lead their effort and provide them with valuable suggestions and insights.[15]

The Nurses' Coalition for Action in Politics (N-CAP) is in the process of establishing a Congressional District network to serve as the "eyes and ears" of N-CAP at the Congressional District level.[16] N-CAP's goal is to have an organization in every Congressional District in the United States. The network is being developed by Congressional District Coordinators who will:

1. provide N-CAP with political, socioeconomic, media and health related data about the Congressional District;
2. identify important geographic subunits within the Congressional District;
3. identify major employers of nurses in each Congressional District;
4. recruit a coordinator in each work place.[17]

Nurses involved in N-CAP's network will benefit too. They will become known to politicians in their Congressional Districts; gain political skills; and get to know N-CAP leadership as well as greater numbers of nurses in their Congressional Districts.

Another example of political networking in action has occurred at the University of Virginia's School of Nursing. A legislative awareness task force has been established at the school to assist faculty and students to become aware of and involved in the legislative process, to gather and disseminate legislative information, and to contact organizations involved in influencing legislation. The purposes were accomplished by placing task force members in the school lobby at specified times to provide legislative information, by holding a legislative awareness day, and by conducting voter registration drives.[18]

The "old boys'" and "old girls'" networks can work together to influence politicians. Such a combination of networks can result in effective coalitions. In Indiana, optometrists, pharmacists, nurses, podiatrists, and psychologists have worked through their organizations in a loosely organized coalition, now over 10 years old, to influence members of the Indiana General Assembly on a variety of issues. Members of the coalition exchange information on a routine basis about such issues as credentialing, continuing education, and third-party reimbursement.

Prior to the general elections in Indiana, the Indiana Optometric Association conducts a series of prelegislative dinners around the state to which candidates for state legislature are invited. Coalition members also are invited. Subsequently, select members of the Indiana State Nurses' Association attend these dinners. This is a great opportunity for these nurses to network with politicians and other health care professionals and to develop a larger network for themselves and for their professional association.

Political networks, like other networks, are kept alive by care and feeding. As an individual you can do a great deal to keep your personal, political network alive and well. You can join and actively support organizations that have viable legislative or political action programs. You can keep up to date on legislative or political issues in nursing by reading various professional journals or attending legislative seminars or political action workshops. You can continuously monitor events and changes in your network and put them to good advantage.

For example, a legislator you know may have a great interest in exploring alternatives to in-patient hospital care. You will enhance your relationship with this legislator by providing him or her with articles, position statements, or access to information about such things as home care or hospice care. You may even want to escort the legislator on a visit to a hospice or home care agency. The networks you have developed among your colleagues can be of great help in developing a political network. Let's say you met the executive director of the Visiting Nurses' Association (VNA) in your community at a recent continuing education offering. What better way to network than to arrange with the VNA head to bring the chairman of the Senate Public Health Committee (a legislator you know) to the VNA for a visit. The legislator has access to an expert in home care and the executive director of the VNA has met an elected official who may well influence the VNA's operation. The payoff for you is that you have strengthened your network by providing others the opportunity to strengthen and expand their networks.

In another example, a legislator you know has a daughter who wants to be a nurse and asks you to talk with her about the various nursing education programs. If you feel well enough informed to tackle the request on your own, great. If not, contact several of your colleagues who have graduated from two-, three-, and four-year programs in nursing to meet with you and the legislator's daughter to discuss the various education options. The state board of nursing can be contacted for a list of schools of nursing operating in your state. Again, you are networking for political impact.

In still another example, your precinct committeeman wants to make a career change. He is considering nursing but does not know if the nursing profession or caring for the ill is for him. He asks for your advice. In this instance, you will want to call upon your network to provide the committeeman with several opportunities. You might put the committeeman in touch with the volunteer services at the local hospital in order that he might have the opportunity to experience an environment in which people are ill. Also, you will want to arrange for the committeeman to see a career counselor at a school of nursing in your area.

SUMMARY

Developing political skills and contacts will provide many opportunities to participate in decision making about societal resources and their allocation. As a networker, your contacts and skills in the political arena will help you get ahead but you also will be called upon to return favors and to help others advance, personally or professionally. Being called upon for assistance by those in your political network is a recognition of your power and influence.

NOTES

1. Carolyne K. Davis et al., "Leadership for Expanding Nursing Influence on Health Policy," *The Journal of Nursing Administration*, January 1982, p. 1.

2. Beatrice J. Kalisch and Philip A. Kalisch, *Politics of Nursing* (Philadelphia: Lippincott, 1982), p. xi.

3. Marjorie Stanton, "Political Action and Nursing," *Nursing Clinics of North America* (Philadelphia: Saunders, 1974), p. 579.

4. Shirley Fondiller, ed., "U.S. Congress Overrides Veto of HEW Funding," *The American Nurse* 8, no. 3 (March 1976): 1.

5. New Hampshire Nurses Association, "Legislative Update," *Nursing News* 31, no. 8 (December 1981): 1.

6. Thelma Schorr, ed., "Nurses Politically Concerned and Active Study of Voting Habits Reveals," *American Journal of Nursing* 79, no. 7 (July 1979): 1181–1196.

7. American Nurses' Association, "N-CAP Develops Grass-Roots Structure To Help 'Deliver' Nursing's Vote," *The Political Nurse* 1, no. 6 (December 1981): 1.

8. Kalisch and Kalisch, *Politics of Nursing*, p. 367.

9. Conversation with Loretta Graf, Member, Board of Trustees, Nurses' Coalition for Action in Politics, June 7, 1982.

10. American Nurses' Association, "Don't Just Stand There, Run!" *The Political Nurse* 1, no. 5 (October 1981): 3.

11. American Nurses' Association, "Political Update," *The Political Nurse* 2, no. 1 (February 1982): 1.

12. Davis, *The Journal of Nursing Administration*, p. 17.

13. Billye C. Pearson, "Legislators Hear Voice of Nursing Network," *AORN Journal* 30, no. 4 (October 1979): 782–786.

14. Indiana State Nurses' Association, "Plan for ISNA Member/State Legislator Communications Network," July 1980, p. 1.

15. American Nurses' Association, "New Hampshire Nurses Learn Politics the Hard Way," *The Political Nurse* 2, no. 2 (April 1982): 1.

16. American Nurses' Association, "N-CAP Develops Grass-Roots Structure To Help 'Deliver' Nursing's Vote," p. 10.

17. Ibid., p. 1.

18. Patricia A. Powell and Parry J. Knauss, "The Legislative Task Force: A Method To Increase Nurses' Political Involvement," *Nursing Outlook* 29, no. 12 (December 1981): 715–716.

Chapter 6

Applying Networking to Labor Relations

Linda J. Shinn

As noted in Chapter 2, many nurses are neither aware of how decisions are made in their employment setting nor of how they could work to affect those decisions being made. This chapter will focus on the utilization of the interdependent network of relationships that exist in the employment setting for professional and personal benefit. The chapter will further explore the forging of alliances in the employment setting in an attempt to establish and strengthen working relationships.

NURSING AND LABOR RELATIONS

Historically, registered nurses have turned to collective bargaining to make a difference in their terms and conditions of employment. In 1946, for example, the American Nurses' Association inaugurated an economic security program. It was hoped that the program would "stabilize nursing services, improve working conditions and provide immediate and long term economic security for nurses in all fields of employment. State nurses' associations were urged to conduct active programs, including collective bargaining, for nurses."[1]

Another example of networking in nursing to improve terms and conditions of employment occurred in the mid-60s. At that time, the American Nurses' Association's House of Delegates adopted a salary goal. The Association in essence said that the basic beginning salary for a person entering the profession of nursing should be $6,500.

Subsequently, the network of state nurses' associations followed suit. For example, the Florida Nurses' Association reported that adoption of the salary goal and informing nurse employers about the salary goal was in itself enough to bring about some increases in pay. Utah also supported the salary goal, as did North Carolina, North Dakota, Texas, and Nebraska.[2]

In the late 60s and early 70s, it was not unusual for nurse employers to call state nurses' associations to find out what recommended salaries were. Many directors of nursing reported that such a salary goal was helpful to them in articulating a good case for increased salaries in nursing budgets.

The setting of salary goals is no longer done by the American Nurses' Association or its constituent state associations. Such a practice can be construed as price fixing and a violation of federal antitrust laws.

In the 70s, particularly since the 1974 amendment of the National Labor Relations Act to permit collective bargaining among health care workers in the private, nonprofit health care setting, organizing for the purposes of collective bargaining has become another route by which nurses are establishing networks to improve the terms and conditions of their employment. In 1976, the American Hospital Association reported that, among member hospitals surveyed, 23 percent had at least one collective bargaining agreement with a labor organization. That is in contrast to 16 percent in 1970.[3] Many labor organizations view the health care industry as "ripe" for organizing and a great untapped resource for union memberships.

The use of the collective bargaining tool has become a very popular way to make an impact on terms and conditions of employment in health care work settings. Collective bargaining in these settings seems here to stay.

How then should nurses prepare themselves to respond to the utilization of the collective bargaining technique to influence terms and conditions of employment? In other words, what networks can be forged to help staff nurses or nursing service administrators positively influence the employment environment?

LABOR RELATIONS TERMINOLOGY

One of the first things that needs to be done is to understand some of the "jargon" or terminology that is used in labor relations circles. The following are definitions of commonly used terms in labor relations:

- *Agreement*—The written instrument that sets forth the results of negotiations. Generally, the agreement contains such items as salary schedules, benefit packages, grievance procedures, and procedures by which nurses, for example, can participate in influencing patient care in the practice setting.
- *Arbitration*—The submission of a dispute between employer and employee to an impartial third party called an arbitrator. Arbitration is voluntary when the parties to a dispute agree to submit the dispute

to an impartial third party. Compulsory arbitration is arbitration required by law. Arbitration can result in recommendations by the arbitrator that are advisory to or binding upon the parties in a dispute.

- *Authorization Card*—A document signed by an employee that authorizes an organization to represent the employee in dealings with an employer over wages, hours, and working conditions.

- *Bargaining Unit*—A group of employees found to be appropriate for representation in the collective bargaining process. The unit can be designated by a labor board or agreed upon by an employer and the employee organization.

- *Boycott*—The collaboration among organizations or groups of people in the avoidance of a particular product made by a particular industry. The refusal to purchase or handle a specific product also constitutes a boycott.

- *Collective Bargaining*—The negotiation of wages, hours, and working conditions.

- *Comparable Worth*—The equation of wages and salaries; concept in the nursing profession that has resulted in efforts by registered nurses to seek wages or salaries equal to health professionals with like backgrounds and responsibilities in the same geographic locale.

- *Decertification*—When a labor organization loses its recognition as the exclusive bargaining agent for a group of employees, or when an agency, such as the National Labor Relations Board, withdraws certification upon certain conditions, such as a majority vote by the employees desiring the withdrawal of official recognition or certification.

- *Deficit Financing*—A provision found in many contracts between public employers and public employee representatives that requires that governmental units not negotiate contract provisions requiring monies that exceed those available to the governmental unit.

- *Dues Deduction*—Money withheld from the paycheck of a member of a labor organization or other group that is used to pay the member's dues to the labor organization or other membership agency.

- *Election*—An election conducted by a particular governmental agency to determine whether or not employees wish to be represented for the purposes of collective bargaining. Usually termed a representation election.

- *Exclusive Representative*—An employee organization certified by an agency such as the National Labor Relations Board or recognized by the employer as the representative of employees for the purposes of collective bargaining.

- *Factfinding*—The gathering of data about a dispute, including the positions of the parties to the dispute and the recommendation of a settlement of the dispute by the factfinders. Factfinders are individuals designated to investigate and report the facts about a dispute; factfinders may have authority to recommend a resolution to the dispute.

- *Federal Mediation and Conciliation Service (FMCS)*—An agency of the federal government that makes mediators available to assist parties in dispute to reach a settlement. The FMCS also can be called upon to provide rosters of arbitrators.

- *Final Offer*—A process whereby parties to an impasse each submit a final offer to a third party. The third party selects the most reasonable offer, which becomes binding on each party to the dispute. Final offer provisions are found in several public employee collective bargaining statutes.

- *Grievance*—An employee complaint about an employment condition or the interpretation or application of a contract provision.

- *Grievance Procedure*—A formalized process, via a contract or personnel policies, that provides a step-by-step mechanism for adjusting employee complaints. The first step of the grievance procedure usually begins with an informal discussion with the employee's immediate supervisor. The final step may be arbitration.

- *Impasse*—When parties to contract negotiations reach a point at which differences cannot be resolved by continued bargaining.

- *Job Posting*—The announcement of job openings by the posting of notices on a bulletin board in the employment setting. Job posting, often provided for in a contract, may give employees the opportunity for promotion or job reassignment.

- *Labor Organization*—An organization that has as one of its purposes or functions the representation of employees for influencing wages, hours, and working conditions, usually via collective bargaining. Among the labor organizations representing nurses are the American Nurses' Association; the Federation of Nurses and Health Professionals, American Federation of Teachers, AFL-CIO; the American Federation of State, County and Municipal Employees, AFL-CIO; and 1199, the National Union of Hospital and Health Care Employees International Union, AFL-CIO, and the Teamsters.

- *Mediation*—A third party aids in the resolution of an impasse between employer and employee.

- *National Labor Relations Act (NLRA)*—A federal law that sets forth the parameters for the participation of employers and employees in industry and the nonpublic health care setting in the collective bargaining process.
- *National Labor Relations Board (NLRB)*—A federal agency established to administer the National Labor Relations Act. The Board, with headquarters in Washington, D.C., has regional offices throughout the country.
- *Negotiations*—The coming together of two parties, usually the employer and employee representative, to discuss, debate, and compromise on the subject matter at hand, usually terms and conditions of employment.
- *Negotiating Team*—A group of individuals representing management or a labor organization who discuss, debate, and compromise on terms and conditions of employment, resulting in an agreement.
- *No Lockout Clause*—A contract provision wherein the employer agrees not to lock employees out of the work setting for the duration of a contract. This clause usually is coupled with a no strike clause.
- *No Strike Clause*—A contract provision wherein the employees agree not to strike. This clause usually is coupled with a no lockout clause.
- *Public Employee Collective Bargaining Statute*—A state, county, or municipal law that sets forth the rules by which employers and employees at the state or local level of government may engage in collective bargaining.
- *Public Law 95-454*—A federal statute that regulates collective bargaining in federal sector employment. It also is referred to as the Federal Employment Labor Management Relations Statute. It sets forth the guidelines for collective bargaining in the federal governmental sector.
- *Professional Performance Committee (PPC)*—A committee of bargaining unit members created to discuss and recommend to or advise management on issues related to patient care, such as staffing, equipment needs, and so on. Similar committees may be negotiated in contracts under the title "Advisory Committee," "Unit/Management Cooperation Committee," "Staffing Advisory Committee," and the like.
- *Ratification*—The approval of a contract by employees affected by the contract.
- *R.N. Unit*—A group of registered nurses in a particular employment setting who have come together to improve wages, hours, and working conditions. (May be referred to as the "local unit.")

- *Right to Work Law*—A statute forbidding the negotiation of contract language that requires employees to become members of a labor organization.
- *Steward (Unit or Area Representative)*—A labor organization member whose duties include assisting union members in adjusting grievances, transmitting information, collecting union dues, and recruiting new union members.
- *Strike*—A lawful or unlawful work stoppage, absence from work, or failure to perform work by employees in a concerted manner in an effort to slow down or shut down the operation of the employer.
- *Supervisor*—A person who has the authority over employees or groups of employees to hire, fire, transfer, suspend, lay off, recall, reward, promote, assign, or discipline them or to effectively recommend such action. Definitions set forth in various statutes usually describe a supervisor as one whose duties in relation to other employees require the use of independent judgment, not just the carrying out of routine work or clerical skills.
- *Unfair Labor Practice*—An action by the employer or employee group that violates provisions of labor law. An example of an unfair labor practice is an employer's refusal to bargain in good faith with the certified representative of the employees.
- *Union Security Clause*—A contract provision that regulates employees' membership in a union. Such a provision generally is written to require an employee to belong to a labor organization during the life of a contract, to maintain employment, or to pay equal to or greater than union dues if the employee does not wish to join the union. Lack of a specific membership provision in a contract sets the stage for an employee to join or refrain from joining the labor organization.

RUDIMENTS OF LABOR LAW

If you become involved in collective bargaining as a member of the nursing staff or as a member of the nursing management team, it is extremely important that you be familiar with the rudiments of labor law. The following discussion of labor law is not intended to be comprehensive but to highlight some important points in the National Labor Relations Act, the Federal Service Labor Management Relations Statute (Public Law 95-454), and a sample public employee collective bargaining statute at the state level. An in-depth review of any of the aforementioned laws should be undertaken if more detailed information is desired.

Single complimentary copies of the Federal Service Labor Management Relations Statute or the National Labor Relations Act may be obtained from members of the U.S. Congress, purchased from the U.S. Government Printing Office, or read at the local library.

Federal Service Labor Management Relations Statute

Public Law 95-454 is applicable to those employed by the federal government, such as nurses employed by the Veteran's Administration. This statute, administered by a three-member Federal Labor Relations Authority, provides federal employees the right to form or join a labor organization or to refrain from doing so. The statute gives federal employees the right to engage in collective bargaining over certain terms and conditions of employment.

The law contains a number of definitions. For example, a supervisor is defined as one who has the authority, generally, to hire and fire. The supervisory definition further specifies that a nursing supervisor is one who devotes a preponderance or majority of employment time to supervisory duties. Supervisors cannot be represented for collective bargaining, nor can they be members of the bargaining unit.

The definition section also defines a professional employee as a person who has advanced knowledge as a result of studying in an institution of higher education or a hospital and who consistently exercises discretion or judgment in the work or practice setting. Also, the professional individual's work must be predominantly intellectual in nature and neither routinized nor standardized. Registered nurses are professional employees under this statute and do have the right to participate in all professional bargaining units.

A labor organization that desires to represent a group of federal employees, such as nurses, must demonstrate that it has a 30 percent showing of interest among those employees who wish to be represented for the purposes of collective bargaining. The Federal Labor Relations Authority may conduct a hearing to determine the membership of a bargaining unit.

An election usually is held among the members of the bargaining unit to determine if employees want to be represented for the purposes of collective bargaining. A majority of those who vote in the election determine the election outcome, in other words, whether or not there will be collective bargaining in a particular work setting. Should the employees select not to be organized for the purposes of collective bargaining, the Authority will not conduct another election for the unit for 12 months.

A labor organization representing federal employees is obligated to represent all members of the bargaining unit whether or not the employee is a member of the labor organization. Negotiable items in the federal sector include such matters as a grievance procedure, payroll dues deduction, and conditions of employment, such as personnel policies and practices not provided for in federal statute or regulations.

Negotiations over budgetary items, such as salary and fringe benefits, usually are not possible in the federal sector as these matters are determined by the U.S. Congress or other federal agencies. Strikes, work stoppages, or slowdowns also are prohibited by the statute. The Federal Mediation and Conciliation Service is required to participate in the resolution of impasses that might occur in negotiations.

National Labor Relations Act

The National Labor Relations Act (NLRA) is administered by the National Labor Relations Board (NLRB) and protects the right of employees in private sector employment to organize and bargain collectively. The definition section of the act also defines "supervisor" as one having the authority to hire and fire, although no reference is made to nurses per se in this definition. "Professional employee" as defined in the NLRA is quite similar to the definition embodied in the Federal Service Labor Management Relations Statute. The term "health care institution" as defined in the NLRA includes "any hospital, convalescent hospital, health maintenance organization, health clinic, nursing home, extended care facility or other institution devoted to the care of the sick, infirm or aged persons."[4]

Employees in the private for-profit and private nonprofit sector of employment can organize for the purposes of collective bargaining or refrain from doing so under the NLRA except in those instances in which an agreement has been negotiated requiring membership in a labor organization as a condition of employment. Membership requirements in a labor organization are negotiable items under the NLRA.

Other negotiable items include wages, hours of work, grievance procedures, and other terms and conditions of employment. Items commonly negotiated in nurses' contracts include schedule posting, provisions regarding part-time employment and staff relief, inservice education, professional performance committees, on-call pay, and shift pay differentials and wages.

Under the NLRA, professional employees also have the opportunity to establish a bargaining unit that does not include nonprofessional workers. Moreover, a majority of the votes cast determines the election outcome in the private sector. Further, no election can be conducted in a unit in which there has been an election in a prior 12-month period.

While mandatory membership is a negotiable item under the National Labor Relations Act, any employee of a health care institution who is a member of a particular religious sect that has historically objected to the support of a labor organization engaged in collective bargaining is not required to become and remain a labor organization member. This particular individual can, however, be required to pay a sum equal to the dues amount to a nonreligious charitable fund. This fund also is a negotiable matter.

Strikes are permissible under the NLRA and the act sets forth certain notice requirements that must be followed prior to striking. In the health care industry, a 60- to 90-day notice requirement of the existence of a dispute is required prior to taking a strike action. In addition, the Federal Mediation and Conciliation Service is required to communicate with the parties involved and attempt to mediate the dispute and bring about some agreement.

Both statutes described above contain fairly extensive unfair labor practice sections applicable to the employer and employee representative. Unfair labor practices might include such acts as interference in an employee organizaton by management and management coercion of employees in exercising their rights to participate or not to participate in bargaining. Unfair labor practices applicable to employee organizations can include discrimination in terms of membership in the labor organization, refusal to bargain, and coercion of an employer in the selection of bargaining representatives.

State Public Sector Collective Bargaining Statutes

According to O'Rourke and Barton, 22 states have public sector collective bargaining laws.[5] These laws vary a great deal in content and coverage. Generally, the coverage section of the statute will define those public employees who have the right to organize for collective bargaining and those who are not accorded this privilege. For example, Indiana has a public employee collective bargaining law that covers public school teachers only. Some states have collective bargaining statutes that protect state employees only; other state laws include state, county, and municipal workers.

Public sector laws usually have a definition section that will, more than likely, include a definition of supervisor similar to that in the NLRA and the Federal Labor Management Relations Act. Public employee statutes frequently will contain a definition of professional employee and accord the professional worker the right to establish a professional bargaining unit.

Public sector bargaining units may be quite large. It is not unusual for a bargaining unit of professional state employees to include, for example, all employees employed by state-supported colleges or universities or all employees employed in state hospitals. In public sector employment, a state collective bargaining statute might provide for collective bargaining to take place between the public employer and public employee representative or it might provide for only a "meet and confer" type of arrangement. In other words, in the latter instance, the employer is required to meet and discuss employment issues with the representative of public employees but the terms and conditions of employment do not have to be reduced to writing, nor is there any vehicle or mechanism to enforce the outcome of the discussions.

Negotiable items at the state level vary. In some instances, terms and conditions of employment, including salaries and benefits, are negotiable items. In other instances, salary ranges and salary increments, benefits, and personnel classifications are not negotiable as they are issues decided upon by state legislatures, governors, or other state governmental agencies.

Mandating membership requirements in the labor organization varies from state to state. In "right to work" states, no membership security arrangements may be negotiated in collective bargaining agreements. In some states, a maintenance of membership or union shop clause is negotiable.

Strikes usually are prohibited under state statutes. However, strikes have occurred among public sector employees, most notably among the teacher groups. Most public sector collective bargaining statutes will prescribe penalties for the breaking of the strike prohibition. Such penalties range from heavy fines, prison terms, and loss of employment to loss of union recognition and dues deduction privileges.

Often, public sector statutes will set forth certain requirements for the resolution of a dispute or an impasse during negotiations. Mediation, factfinding, arbitration, or final offer selection are among the options to settle disputes or impasses.

County/Local Level Collective Bargaining Laws

In some states, employees at the county or municipal levels of government are covered under state statutes or under local ordinances that permit collective bargaining or meeting and conferring with the local-level public employer. Local public employees to which local- or state-level statutes are applicable may include sanitation and parks department workers, municipal or county hospital employees, and employees of public health departments.

Among the negotiable items at the local level are wages, benefits, and grievance procedures. Strikes usually are prohibited.

DECIDING WHETHER OR NOT TO ORGANIZE

" . . . [o]nly poor administrative practices drive nurses into unions."[6] More often than not, registered nurses are driven to organizing for the purposes of collective bargaining because of poor communications or poor networks in the employment settings. If registered nurses are not an integral part of the employment network, kept abreast of changes in policies and procedures, kept aware of decisions made by administrators and nursing managers, and given the opportunity to have a voice in decisions made or changes contemplated, then nurses will seek a mechanism whereby they can force themselves into the decision-making network in the employment setting. Often, the mechanism selected is collective bargaining.

The following examples illustrate reasons given by groups of nurses for organizing:

- Small Midwestern Hospital

Nurses were required to run the pharmacy from 5 P.M. until 7 A.M. In the meantime, evening and night nurse/patient staffing ratios were at an all-time low. Nurses became very irate at serving as the "pharmacist" in addition to doing other nonnursing functions and, thus, having fewer resources to devote to the practice of nursing. Subsequently, these nurses sought help from a state nurses' association in rectifying this situation and ultimately organized for collective bargaining.

- Large Eastern Nursing Home

A nursing home administrator publicly announced that his policy was to practice "thin" staffing. As a result, when nurses resigned or retired, they were not replaced. As the number of staff decreased, the patient load for nurses increased, weekends off decreased, and the necessity to rotate shifts increased. Nurses turned to a union and organized.

- Large Western Hospital

Lack of adequate orientation and training for nurses working in specialty units and inadequate supervision of nonnursing personnel resulted in nurse employees seeking the help of a labor organization.

Exhibit 6–1 Sample Facility Grievance Procedure

Step 1.	An employee having a complaint about the terms or conditions of employment or who feels he/she has been dealt with unfairly at Hyde Hospital should discuss those complaints or concerns with his/her immediate supervisor. Should the employee feel that the concerns are not adequately addressed by the immediate supervisor in 10 calendar days, the employee should proceed to Step 2.
Step 2.	The complaint or concern should be documented in writing and given to the Department Head. (For example, registered nurses should transmit their grievances to the Director of Nursing.) The Department Head shall respond to the employee's grievance in writing within 10 calendar days of the receipt of the grievance.
Step 3.	If the employee is not satisfied with the response of the Department Head, the employee may forward his/her complaint in writing to the Director of the Personnel Department. The Director of the Personnel Department will have 7 calendar days from the date of receipt of the grievance to respond to the employee's grievance in writing.
Step 4.	If the employee is not satisfied with the response to the complaint by the Director of the Personnel Department, the employee may address his/her grievance in writing to the Hospital Administrator. The Hospital Administrator shall respond to the aggrieved employee in writing within 7 calendar days of receipt of the complaint. The Hospital Administrator's decision shall be final and binding.

On occasion, other options are exercised by nurses in lieu of organizing for the purpose of collective bargaining. Such options have included addressing problems through the facility's grievance procedure. In many instances, nurses are not aware that a grievance procedure exists in the job setting although a grievance procedure usually is contained in the personnel policies. Sometimes, utilizing this procedure will resolve problems. A sample facility grievance procedure appears as Exhibit 6-1.

On occasion, nurses get together as a group and discuss their problems and potential solutions and, if the employer "gets wind" of such a meeting, concerns may be taken care of. Some nurses will use the strategy of inviting a labor organization representative to meet with them in order to indirectly pressure management to attend to their concerns.

For example, one group of nurses in a tiny, rural hospital had no lockers for coats or other personal belongings. The employer had been pestered for years by these nurses to find locker space for the employees. Subsequently, the nurses held a mass meeting to which they invited all hospital employees and a representative of a labor organization. New lockers were in place by the start of the day shift the morning following the meeting with the labor organization representative.

Once in a while, nurses will circulate petitions among colleagues and other employees to protest or urge a particular course of action. Again, changes have been brought about using such a strategy.

NETWORKING DURING THE ORGANIZING PROCESS

If collective bargaining has been selected as the route to address problems in a particular employment setting, networking can be a great aid to the organizational process. Often two or three nurses will be discussing their concerns about the work environment and how to make some changes. Subsequently, these nurses each talk to another colleague and, suddenly, there are six nurses concerned about what is happening on the job. They may meet over coffee in someone's home or for lunch on a day off and discuss ways to deal with their problems.

Frequently, one of the nurses will suggest calling a labor organization such as the state nurses' association for guidance. This potential representative of these nurses may encourage them to use their already established networks or contacts in the employment setting to interest other nurses in a meeting of those who would be eligible for participation in collective bargaining. Word-of-mouth or one-to-one contact may result in a large group of nurses from the facility attending a meeting to discuss the mechanics and legalities of organizing.

An exchange to start the ball rolling, at a fictitious hospital named Saint Paul's, might go something like this:

> *Jane:* I'm so frustrated. If I have to spend one more shift attempting to orient new personnel to my unit and at the same time be responsible for 40 patients, supervising 3 aides, and answering the questions of 10 nursing students attempting to select patients for tomorrow's clinical, I'll explode.
> *Linda:* I know. It seems like they hire people off the street, bring them in and think they can be of immediate assistance to us on our units. It's almost more dangerous than not having enough staff.
> *Jane:* I get nowhere talking to my supervisor about my concerns. She doesn't listen.

Linda: Let's call the state nurses' association and see whether or not they might help us.

Jane: Great! I will talk to Sandy, Denise, and Barbara; they've expressed similar concerns. Maybe they would like to get together with us when we talk to the state nurses' association.

After the state nurses' association has been contacted, Jane and Linda would like to get a larger group of nurses together to meet with the state nurses' association representative to discuss collective bargaining. Jane and Linda decide to meet after work with Sandy, Denise, and Barbara to discuss how to contact other nurses.

At the meeting, all agree they will be responsible for making one non-supervisory contact on each of three units. They divide up the nursing units on which they are to make their contacts.

Subsequently, fifteen contacts are made and each individual contacted is asked to mention to other nurse colleagues the date, time, and place of a meeting to be held to discuss some of the problems in the employment setting. A network of nurses has been born. Thirty-two nurses attend the meeting with the labor representative from the state nurses' association.

At this meeting, rudiments of labor law and labor and legal terminology are discussed. The pros and cons of collective bargaining are explored.

The nurses express concern about what organizing might mean in terms of relationships with one another, with nursing service administrators, hospital administration, the hospital board of trustees, and the community. The state nurses' association representative suggests that the nurses be in touch with several other organized facilities in the community to find out how nurses in those facilities coped with organizing and the problems involved in the organizing process.

Jane remarks that she attends church with a nurse who works at Heritage Hospital and the nurses at Heritage Hospital are organized. Jane offers to talk with her church friend about her experience at Heritage Hospital. Denise reports that one of the members of her Jazzercise class works for City Hospital, where the nurses also are organized. Denise offers to make a contact with the City Hospital nurse. Both Jane and Denise are calling upon the networks they have already built for help.

Denise's contact might go like this:

Denise: Freida, may I talk with you for a minute before class starts?
Freida: Sure.

Denise: We have been discussing organizing for collective bargaining at the hospital where I work. We really need to know more about it; not so much how it actually works, but what it means in terms of changes in the institution, what can be expected in terms of outcome, and what can be anticipated in terms of management's response to us. I understand at City Hospital the registered nurses are organized and have a contract with the hospital. Can you tell me a little bit about your experience in the process of getting organized and negotiating a contract?

Freida: Collective bargaining at City is a little bit different than it is in the private sector. The things we can negotiate for are different from the things you might be able to negotiate at your hospital. For example, we can't negotiate much in terms of wages and benefits but one of the plusses for us has been the opportunity to get to know one another better and to have a forum for discussion of our problems. When we have a problem, according to our contract, we can take that problem to the chief nurse at the monthly meetings that occur between the chief and our local unit chairperson. The local unit representatives submit an agenda for the meeting to the chief and we have found if we prepare our case well and have adequate data to back up our concerns that we often get those concerns taken care of. The local unit has become a good network for nurses in our setting to discuss mutual problems and to exchange information. The unit has also helped us establish a network with the nurse managers at City.

Jane's contact might proceed as follows:

Jane: We are discussing organizing for collective bargaining at the hospital where I work and I wondered if you might be able to tell me about your experiences at Heritage Hospital?

Heritage Hospital Friend: For us, it has been an uphill battle. Management really resisted our organizing and refused to come to the bargaining table for a long time after our unit was organized and the state nurses' association was certified as our bargaining agent. Of course, Heritage was the first hospital to be organized in the state after the laws were changed to permit health care workers in the private nonprofit sector to organize. I'm sure there was a lot of pressure on the administration and others to keep us from being organized and setting any kind of a precedent.

At any rate, we didn't get everything we wanted in our contract. We got a 7 percent salary increase. We finally have a retirement program and that is certainly of benefit to all of us and it's something we didn't have before. We have the opportunity through our professional performance committee to come together on a regular basis to discuss concerns about care of patients at the hospital.

The information gathered by Jane and Denise is taken back to the others and it is agreed that a meeting of all registered nurses interested in organizing should be called and that Denise and Jane's friends should be asked to speak at the meeting and talk with interested nurses about their organizing experiences. In other words, networking among the networks is planned.

Should the nurses in the above example decide to organize, they will want to formalize their networks by establishing a local unit. Also, they will want to adopt a set of bylaws to govern the operation of their local unit and to elect leaders to head their alliance.

An organizing drive will be undertaken by these nurses to solicit the support of all nonsupervisory registered nurses in the hospital to sign authorization cards. See Exhibit 6-2 for a sample authorization card.

The most effective way to recruit or gather support of nurses in the institution will be by using already established contacts to pass the word about the effort being attempted. Personal contact, one to one, one to two, small group meetings, coffees, and informational sessions with labor organization representatives on off-duty time will be used to gather support.

Should a petition be filed with the National Labor Relations Board to take jurisdiction in the instance of Saint Paul's Hospital and an appropriate bargaining unit determined, an election campaign will ensue. Such a campaign is waged by the employer and the employee organization to attempt to influence nurses to vote in support of or against being organized for collective bargaining.

Election campaigns can be very intense. Often, the information that is exchanged during the election process is questionable and may generate fear in the nursing population. The campaign, however, is another good opportunity to make use of a well-functioning nursing network. An operable network through which nurses can keep in constant touch with one another, through which facts can be disseminated and information validated, is very valuable in determining the outcome of the election. A local unit may disseminate information about the campaign by forming a telephone network whereby the local unit officers are each responsible for calling a certain number of members of the local unit to answer questions,

Exhibit 6–2 Authorization card

```
                        AUTHORIZATION CARD


        Indiana State Nurses' Association, 2915 North High School Road
                    Indianapolis, Indiana 46224

        I, _____
            (print)     LAST           First           Middle


        _____
            street & number          City      State      Zip

        do hereby authorize the Indiana State Nurses' Association to be my
        sole and exclusive representative with my employer for the purposes
        of collective bargaining and for all matters concerning rates of
        pay, hours of work and other terms and conditions of employment and
        revoke all other authorizations.

        Employer: _____
                    (name of hospital, agency or institution)

        Address: _____
                    street & number   City      State      Zip

        Indiana R.N. License No. _____S.S. #_____

        Date: _____ Signature: _____
```

Source: Indiana State Nurses' Association, Authorization Card. Reprinted with permission of the Indiana State Nurses' Association.

to give information, and to ensure that people turn out to vote in the election. Exhibit 6-3 displays a sample telephone tree.

The local unit network also is a good forum for monitoring unfair labor practices committed by the employer that may influence the outcome of the election. Such unfair labor practices might include promising favors to employees if they vote against the labor organization in the representation election, raising the wages of those eligible for participation in the bargaining unit, or firing employees for participating in the labor organization activities.

The National Labor Relations Board will be responsible for conducting an election at Saint Paul's Hospital to determine if the nurses want to be represented for collective bargaining and who they want to represent them. Most likely, the election will be conducted on hospital property at a specified date and time.

NEGOTIATIONS, CONTRACT IMPLEMENTATION, STRIKES

Should the election be won by the nurses at Saint Paul's Hospital, negotiating a contract will be next on the nurses' agenda. During the initial

Exhibit 6-3 Local Unit Telephone Tree

Local Unit
Chairperson
777-7777

Local Unit
Vice Chairperson
777-7611

Jane Nelson Telephone Coordinator

Francis Barton	Karen Berg — days
Karen Smith	Paul Coleman — eve.
Rosey Wright	Chuck Stop — nights
Mickey Blue	

Local Unit
Secretary
743-4177

Warren Peach

Peggy Curry	Richy Ball — days
Jean Thomas	Julian Lopaz — eve.
Wilbur Clip	Evan Black — nights
Barry Gale	

Local Unit
Treasurer
729-8900

Pete Nail

Betty Egan	Julie Good — days
Fran Cup	Ann Rule — eve.
Inez Prewitt	Sandy Carr — nights
Bob Stewart	

organizational processes and election campaign, the nurses will have been gathering information about what the nurses in the local unit want included in their negotiated agreement. Members of the local unit may be asked to identify two or three problems of major import to them in the work setting, as well as to recommend solutions for the problems.

Contracts from other organized groups of nurses will be reviewed to see what they contain. Sample copies of other nurses' contracts may be obtained from other local units, from state nurses' associations, and other labor organizations. All of the data collected will be synthesized into contract proposals by the local unit leaders or by the negotiating committee.

The negotiations process is another time during which an effective nursing network vis-à-vis the local unit is important. While not all nurses can participate in negotiations, the negotiating team will want to have the wherewithal to bring proposals back to members of the local unit and to get their input on management's proposals. This can be accomplished through the use of a local unit newsletter, telephone communications system, or local unit meetings.

In an effort to implement a contract, the unit may wish to use, as a matter of practice, stewards or area representatives that serve as liaisons between the nurse and the local unit officers. Such a network also can serve to assist the individual nurse in utilizing the contract. The steward or area representative may help a nurse in pursuing a grievance through the negotiated grievance procedure (Exhibit 6-4) and serve as a conduit between the nurse employee and the local unit officers. The steward or area representative can be a key link in a network established to make a contract work.

On occasion, there is a breakdown in the working relationship between the parties to an agreement. An impasse may result during contract negotiations and, once in a while, the issues are serious enough and important enough to nurses to utilize the strike in an effort to resolve the impasse. A strike is another instance in which an effective, functioning individual and group network is extremely important. Should a strike be selected in an effort to deal with breakdowns in the relationship between the employer and the employee organization, the local unit again serves as the focal point for activities.

Nurses will want to discuss at local unit meetings the pros and cons of a work stoppage and will want to work very closely together to establish the preparations for a strike. Certainly, the communication network to operate during the strike will need to be discussed and established. A telephone tree will be very important for transmitting information in a timely manner.

Exhibit 6–4 Sample Negotiated Grievance Procedure

Article XI.
Preamble: For purposes of this Agreement, a dispute between the parties to the Agreement, Hyde Hospital and Ajax Union, or between Hyde Hospital and a registered nurse covered by this Agreement, concerning the provisions of the Agreement, compliance with or application of the Agreement shall be termed a grievance.

Section 1. Step 1. The nurse shall seek resolution of the grievance with his or her immediate supervisor within 7 calendar days of the event upon which the grievance is based.

Step 2. In the event Step 1 fails the nurse shall have the right to take up the grievance with the Director of Nursing or the designee of the Director of Nursing, either alone or accompanied by a representative of the Ajax Union. The grievance shall be submitted to the Director of Nursing in writing within 14 calendar days of the event upon which the grievance is based. The Director of Nursing or the designee shall meet with the aggrieved to discuss the grievance within 5 calendar days after the grievance has been presented in writing. Within 3 calendar days of the meeting, the Director of Nursing shall respond to the grievance in writing.

Step 3. If the nurse's grievance is not satisfactorily settled at Step 2, the grievance shall be transmitted in writing to the Chief of Employee Relations within 7 working days after the grievance has been answered by the Director of Nursing or the Director's designee. The Chief of Employee Relations, the Director of Nursing or the Director's designee, the grievant and a representative of the Ajax Union shall meet within 5 working days after the grievance has been appealed to the Chief of Employee Relations. The Chief of Employee Relations shall respond to the grievance in writing within 5 working days after the party's last meeting.

Step 4. In the event the grievance is not settled at Step 3 the grievance may be submitted to arbitration by Hyde Hospital or the Ajax Union.

Section 2. The arbitrator shall be selected from a list of arbitrators provided by the Federal Mediation and Conciliation Service. When the list is received the parties shall select an arbitrator by alternately striking names from the list. The party which submitted the grievance to arbitration shall strike first. The arbitrator selected shall conduct a hearing on the grievance within 30 days of the date of selection and shall issue a decision within 30 days of the conclusion of the hearing. The arbitrator shall not modify in any way the terms of the Agreement. The arbitrator's decision shall be final and binding. The cost of arbitration shall be borne equally by the parties to the Agreement.

Section 3. Grievances may be processed during working hours upon the consent of the Hospital and if there is no disruption of patient care services.

The strategies for conducting the strike, the strategies for communicating during a strike, and the strategies for communicating with other labor organizations, with members of the community, and with the media also will need to be worked out. Much of this work, particularly those parts of the puzzle that involve relationships with the media, the community, and other labor organizations, should take place long before a strike is needed. A state nurses' association or any other labor organization representing registered nurses should be able to help guide the local unit in terms of developing media contacts, cultivating relationships, and establishing networks with others. In addition, other nursing units within the community might be called upon for assistance in preparing for and conducting a strike. A strike fund may have been established by the local unit to aid in financing a work stoppage. The strike fund of a labor organization also may be tapped for assistance during the conduct of a strike.

Communications up and down the network established within the local unit are absolutely essential during a strike. The use of written communications through strike bulletins, the use of telephone networks, meetings, rallies, and personal communication is a must to reinforce the transmission of accurate information about what is going on during a work stoppage. A good communications network will help keep all parties together and cohesive, necessary ingredients in a strike situation.

One nurse describes the failure to network during a strike as follows: ". . . we made the classic mistake of not working with the personnel in the hospital, lab techs, maintenance people, X-ray techs, secretaries and so on to get their support. . . . It cost us in lack of support. All these people were crossing our picket lines because they did not even know what our issues were. True, we got moral support from some. But that's not enough."[7]

This same nurse goes on to describe the strike at Woodlawn Park Hospital in Portland, Oregon, as follows: "For us the worst times came when we were picketing alone (we tried to keep the line going 24 hours a day) or when we were at home, away from the other strikers. That's when our imaginations ran wild. The most common nightmare was that each of us was the last one out. We combatted these problems, first by parking a mobile van near the picket site so we could relax and get a cup of coffee, talk. And second by installing a log book in the van where each of us could record our feelings, doubts and fears. That way we reassured each other that our fears were normal. It helped."[8]

DECERTIFICATION

On occasion, nurses find that being organized for collective bargaining is not for them. Subsequently, they decide to decertify their bargaining unit. In essence, the decertification process is much like the initial process to certify the bargaining unit representative. A showing of interest in decertifying the unit is gathered, a decertification petition is filed, a decertification campaign is waged, and a vote is conducted by the appropriate labor board.

One nurse explains the effort to decertify as follows: " . . . using our own funds for printing and postage, we began sending letters to Midland RNs explaining issues and inviting them to come to Joe's house for a series of informal talks over coffee. We had the petitions ready and assured the nurses that coming to one of our parties and signing a petition did not constitute a vote."[9]

Thus, a network was established, perhaps outside the local unit network, in this particular situation to get rid of the bargaining agent. It is quite possible that the hospital involved used all of the resources at its disposal and their networks to assist the network that was being established to decertify the bargaining agent. The nurses, in this instance, apparently did a good job of networking as the vote was 92 to 54 in favor of decertifying.[10]

MANAGEMENT NURSES' NETWORKS

An extensive, functional network among managers, particularly nursing managers, is essential in the employment setting. Clear lines of authority and responsibility, a functional administrative chart, and adequate job descriptions are essential components of the nursing manager's network. Periodic meetings of nurse managers to exchange information, generate new ideas, discuss problems, and hammer out solutions to these problems are essential to maintain the viability of the nursing manager's network.

When the employees that nurses manage organize, it is important that nurse managers have an adequate background in labor law, particularly the laws that govern the employment setting in which they manage, the processes set forth in labor laws that must be followed if employees organize, familiarity with labor terminology, and a good notion of what's going on in the employment setting. Fralic, writing in the *Journal of Nursing Administration,* suggests that the director of nursing needs to be prepared in labor relations matters as follows:

- Know the laws which govern the institution within which he or she manages
- Obtain didactic preparation
- Know terminology
- Keep abreast of labor trends

- Anticipate contract demands
- Know that strikes are the ultimate weapon of the labor organization
- Be a full participant on the negotiating team[11]

Such advice is good for all nursing managers.

The Law

The laws governing the nurse manager's work setting will depend upon whether the facility is public or private. If the facility is public, is it a federal, state, county, or municipal facility? As mentioned previously, private, nonprofit or for-profit health care institutions fall under the jurisdiction of the National Labor Relations Act. If the institution is a public facility operated by the federal government, it will most likely fall under Public Law 95-454. If the agency is a state, county, or municipal agency, local laws will govern. In addition to the sources described earlier in the chapter, copies of the laws should be obtainable from the agency's personnel or legal department. A supply of copies would be a good addition to the nursing manager's library. Among the other laws with which the nurse manager will want to become familiar are:

- wage and hour laws
- occupational safety and health laws
- the Labor Management Reporting and Disclosure Act
- worker's compensation statutes
- applicable hospital or other health care agency licensing laws

Preparation

Academic preparation in labor law or labor management relations generally can be obtained in several ways. Schools of nursing frequently offer graduate preparation in nursing administration that includes labor relations content. Schools of law have labor law courses that can be audited or taken for elective credit. A variety of health care associations and other continuing education providers conduct conferences or workshops on labor law, the "how to" of negotiations, contract enforcement, or grievance processing. Nurse managers are well advised to take advantage of courses or continuing education offerings that provide opportunities for role playing or actual "hands on" practice in negotiations or grievance handling. Such practice will help the nurse manager become more comfortable in applying labor terminology, labor law, negotiations, contract implementation, and grievance techniques.

Terminology and Trends

Many labor relations books define labor terms in further detail than the brief glossary at the beginning of this chapter. In addition, some labor organizations and management associations publish primers on labor terminology.

Regular perusal of literature can be of help to the nurse manager in keeping abreast of trends in the labor management relations arena. Periodicals written specifically for nursing managers, such as the *Journal of Nursing Administration* and *Nursing Management,* frequently carry helpful labor relations information for the nurse manager. Chambers of Commerce usually have Personnel or Labor Relations Departments that publish information about trends in labor relations. Law journals and labor union publications also are good sources of information about trends in labor law and their applications.

Negotiations

Anticipating demands in the negotiation of contracts should not be difficult for nurse managers. If the manager has a "finger on the pulse" of the employment setting, no surprises will arise in contract negotiations. As Fralic points out, problems evident in the employment setting generally surface as subjects for negotiation.[12]

For example, job vacancies in an institution may not be generally advertised to the agency staff. Employees interested in upward mobility or a career change will want to know about positions in the employment setting that are vacant. Subsequently, it can be expected, in a situation where employees are organized or organizing, that the employees will want to negotiate the posting of job vacancies for a specified period of time. Contract language also may be sought that provides employees special consideration in the filling of vacant positions.

Strikes are the ultimate weapon of a labor organization. The right to strike, as noted previously, is permissible in some sectors of employment. Nurse managers should be very familiar with the provisions of labor law that relate to job actions or work stoppages. If a nurse manager anticipates a strike in a particular work setting, he or she may wish to seek advice and counsel from other nurse managers who have experienced a strike. Such contacts can be made through nurse manager networks that have been established among health care facilities in the community, through nurse manager associations or societies, and through labor or legal counsel.

One of nursing's greatest successes over the years has been the garnering of top management positions for nurses in various health care facilities. The struggle of the profession to have qualified nurses named to top administrative posts has been long and arduous, but as a result, many top-flight nursing departments exist throughout the country. The presence and input of the nursing manager is therefore a must in negotiations.

In any negotiations that affect the delivery of patient care, nurse managers must be involved. More often than not, the nursing administrator and other nursing supervisory staff bear the ultimate accountability and responsibility for care given to patients. Authority for decisions made about patient care must be accorded nurse managers to enable them to do their jobs. Thus, it is essential for a nursing manager to be a full participant on any negotiating team when a health care employer enters into collective bargaining with an employee organization. Nurse managers must insist upon involvement in the management network responsible for negotiating conditions under which health care workers are employed and health and nursing care are delivered.

A variety of other links should be built to help nurse managers become effective forces for management in the labor relations arena. Nurse managers should develop ongoing liaison with the person in the facility who is the expert in labor relations, whether it is the personnel director, management consultant, or labor attorney. The expert in labor relations should meet periodically with the nursing managers so that he or she knows what is going on in the facility, what some of the problems are, and, thus, what some of the contract demands are likely to be.

Another component of the manager's network are his or her colleagues in other organized facilities. People who have been through organizing drives, election campaigns, and contract negotiations can be very helpful to nursing managers. These people have firsthand information on how it went, what happened behind the scenes, what can be done to be prepared for collective bargaining in a facility, what kinds of data should be gathered to argue for or against contract proposals, what is required after the contract has been negotiated for the contract to be implemented, how grievance procedures operate, and what can be said to employees about a labor organization and what cannot be said.

Nursing managers should use their networks to plan for and develop strategies to cope with employee work stoppages and strikes. This should include methods for continuing to deliver care and mechanisms for constant communication with the nursing staff remaining on the job, with the negotiating team, the media, and the community, and other health care facilities that might be called upon to assist in delivering patient care or in receiving patients who cannot be cared for in the struck facility.

Once a plan is developed, the nurse manager should readily be able to identify those elements that need to be worked on prior to a strike. Such parts include media relations, community relations, and liaison with other health care facilities in the community. Then the nurse manager can be working with public relations personnel within the facility to forge good media relations and to assist the public relations department to understand on an ongoing basis the issues in delivering patient care. An informed network of contacts and supporters can be very assistive during a strike.

OTHER STRATEGIES

Not all nurses utilize the collective bargaining tool in attempting to influence the terms and conditions of their employment. Other strategies used to influence economic and social conditions in the work setting also require networking.

William Werther and Carol Lockhart, writing in the *Journal of Nursing Administration,* recommend that employers, employees, and employee organizations should cooperate in an effort to generate surplus revenues in the employment setting. Such revenues, they suggest, would lead to more money and benefits for all involved, including health care clients.[13] The "bottom line" would be a more productive, satisfied work force.

While Werther and Lockhart contemplate the use of cooperation in organized employment settings, it seems that collaboration could work in unorganized settings as well. Networking is a natural in establishing a cooperative environment in the employment setting as cooperation can be fostered by individuals, managers, and employees helping one another. Nurse networkers who have developed a system of contacts among their peers, and more than likely enhanced their vertical and horizontal communications channels in the work area, probably have established many cooperative relationships already. These need only be expanded to foster the concept of cooperation in the job setting.

Werther and Lockhart note that the first step to cooperation between an employer and employee group may come when one party needs a favor. "When favors are granted, reciprocation is expected. If they are reciprocated, simple favors and requests for help may slowly create a cooperative relationship."[14]

A number of groups of nurses have used strategies of collective action without collective bargaining to gain mastery over their employment conditions. Again, networking has been involved. For example, the nurses employed by the City of Denver have battled with the city over salary inequities since 1967.[15] They have filed a complaint with the Equal Employment Opportunity Commission and a suit in Federal Court to remedy the pay inequities that have arisen between nurses and other professional public employees, such as sanitarians and civil engineers. Thus far the Denver nurses have regrettably failed to win a remedy for the injustices that exist, but they have experienced dynamic networking in action. It was evident that whatever happened to those nurses in Denver would ricochet around the country and, thus, organized nursing networks like the American Nurses' Association, groups of nurses, and individual nurses contributed human and financial resources to aid the cause of the Denver group.

Other collective action strategies used by nurses include mass sick calls, informational picketing, hand billing, and refusal to do nonnursing duties in the work setting. These approaches to dealing with problems in the employment environment probably have worked best when an informed, organized group of nurses existed. In other words, nurses knew what was going on in the employment setting, who had the power to make changes, and what kind of actions were necessary to influence the change agent. These nurses developed and used contacts and made them work. They networked.

Quality circles have become popular in manufacturing locations and are cropping up in health care delivery settings as well. In essence, quality circles are groups of employees who work in a team with a manager in an effort to improve job quality and the quality of work life.

One condition that nurses have identified in multitudinous surveys is lack of power, influence, or control in the practice setting. It is anticipated that groups of nurses teamed with nursing managers in a quality circle might be one way to eliminate this job dissatisfaction. In many areas nurses can use their problem-solving skills to lead or be an integral part of a team that has the potential to make changes in the work place, to have a voice in the employment setting, to get management's attention, and to be listened to.

The quality circle is another strategy to facilitate employees' involvement in the work area and its success depends heavily on networking. In other words, the basic elements of networking—team work, commitment, and communications—are the essential ingredients for an effective quality circle.

The elements of networking in a quality circle might come into play as follows:

Quality Circle Member: Participating in our quality circle meetings for an hour each week has given me a totally different perspective about my job and my self-worth. It's good to know that I have a forum within which to express my concerns.

Quality Circle Leader: The men and women who staff Creative Hospital are its greatest resource. I'm pleased to be part of the cultivation of this resource. As you know, the topic you recommended for today's agenda is working with the newly graduated nurse at Creative. I recognize we've had a high turnover rate among new grads and a great number of transfer requests from this group of employees. Any suggestions on how we might work together to make their transition from school to work easier on all of us?

Quality Circle Member: I think that our emphasis on teamwork should be extended to the new graduate. We would build a lot of trust, self-worth, and commitment to Creative Hospital if we could institute an RN/new graduate preceptor program. Every new grad hired by Creative should be paired with an RN on the nursing unit for at least 3 to 6 weeks after orientation. This joint venture would permit exchange of information, validation of practice, and an opportunity to get to know the "rules." Also, the new grads should become members of the quality circle as soon as they are hired.

Quality Circle Leader: Other comments or suggestions?

Quality Circle Member: The idea of a preceptor program is a good one. I would have been much more comfortable and sure of myself when I started working here if I could have had one person I could rely on as a sounding board.

Quality Circle Leader: Sounds like the idea is worth a try. I'll talk with the Director of Nursing and Staff Development Coordinator at our weekly meeting scheduled for tomorrow. I'll report back to you next week.

The nurses in the above example have used the quality circle network to recommend the establishment of a new graduate/preceptor network. It appears that a network of staff nurses to nursing managers exists and that persons in authority may be willing to use the ideas from a quality circle as a strategy to improving the well-being of new graduate nurses. Again, dynamic networking in action.

SUMMARY

Whether a member of the nursing staff or nursing management team is involved in collective bargaining, collective action, quality circles, cooperation, or other activities that will influence the work setting, the ability to network effectively is paramount. What you know, who you know, where, when, and how you use the knowledge at your disposal and the contacts you have are the keys to successful networking for nurse managers and members of the nursing staff.

NOTES

1. Lyndia Flannagan, ed., *One Strong Voice: The Story of The American Nurses Association* (Kansas City, Mo.: Lowell Press, 1976), p. 622.

2. Martha Belote, "Nurses Are Making It Happen," *The American Journal of Nursing 67*, no. 2 (February 1967): 286.

3. Beatrice J. Kalisch and Philip A. Kalisch, *Politics of Nursing* (Philadelphia: Lippincott, 1982), p. 397.

4. The National Labor Relations Act, Section 2 (14). *Coverage of Non-profit Hospitals under the National Labor Relations Act,* from U.S. Senate Conference Report no. 93-988, 93rd Congress, 2nd Session, July 8, 1974.

5. Karen O'Rourke and Salley Barton, *Nurse Power, Unions and the Law* (Bowie, Md.: Robert J. Brady Co., 1981), pp. 98–99.

6. Leah Curtin, ed., "Negotiating for a Change," *Supervisor Nurse 11*, no. 9 (September 1980): 7.

7. Patricia S. Chaney, "Protest," *Nursing 77, 7*, no. 2 (February 1977): 26.

8. Ibid.

9. Jan Nantonski, "Why A Union Contract Didn't Work At Our Hospital," *RN Magazine 41*, no. 5 (May 1978): 71.

10. Ibid.

11. Maryann F. Fralic, "The Nursing Director Prepares For Labor Negotiations," *Journal of Nursing Administration 7*, no. 6 (July–August 1977): 5–6.

12. Ibid., p. 5

13. William B. Werther, Jr., and Carol A. Lockhart, "Collective Action and Cooperation in the Health Professions," *Journal of Nursing Administration 7*, no. 6 (July–August 1977): 13.

14. Ibid., p. 18.

15. Patricia S. Chaney, "Protest," p. 30.

Chapter 7

Networking and Other Strategies for Professional Growth

Networking is one strategy that can be used by nurses to attain their professional and personal goals. Networking requires personal and professional abilities and skills. One of the characteristics necessary in order to network expertly is that you know who you are and where you are going (or want to go). One way of determining where you want to go is to establish your personal and professional goals.

Few educational programs that prepare nurses for practice teach them to set professional goals for themselves. Nurses who have set goals for themselves are usually in the minority. Without well-defined and established goals, nurses are left without much direction for their professional careers.

In recent years continuing education courses have included goal setting as part of their content. Generally, these courses are not entirely devoted to professional goal setting, but segments of the content relate to that topic. For example, in a course on nurses as change agents, part of the content may relate to knowing what it is you want in your nursing career (your professional goals) so that you may work to change situations that frustrate your goal achievement. Values clarification and time management workshops also often contain content about setting such goals and meeting them.

CLARIFYING YOUR PROFESSIONAL GOALS

Many individuals have goals, both personal and professional ones, that are more unconscious than conscious. In order to act to achieve your professional goals, you must first understand what they are. If you have been in a situation where you learned to set down your goals in writing, you probably went through the process in several steps.

The first step is to identify the values you hold. Values, as defined by Sidney Simon, noted theorist and practitioner in the area of values clarification, are "a set of personal beliefs and attitudes about the truth, beauty, worth of any thought, object, or behavior. They are action oriented and give direction and meaning to one's life."[1]

Values clarification exercises are useful strategies to clarify one's own values and to see oneself more realistically. When you know who you are and where you are going (or want to go), then you can make choices that will enable you to get there.

One values clarification exercise that is helpful in determining what you value is to place in rank order of importance to you the following items:

- health
- wealth
- responsibility
- prestige
- security
- being a parent
- being a leader
- being famous
- being an expert
- enjoyment of life
- being all you can be
- helping others
- being independent
- serving others

Carefully assessing what is important to you will give you a clearer idea of what your values are.

Next, you can sort out personal (being a parent) from professional (being an expert) values in the previous list. Your professional values may provide you with information helpful in defining your goals. To begin to define your personal and professional goals, respond to the following questions:

- What are some of the things you do well?
- What are some things you don't do well?
- What would you prefer not doing?
- What would you like to start doing?
- What would you like to do more often?

Again, reviewing your responses should reveal some of your interests and values that can be translated into personal and/or professional goals. Knowing who you are and what you want is basic to being able to use strategies such as networking to attain your goals.

Try next to establish your personal and professional goals. Simply list them as they occur to you. Include both short-range goals, which can be accomplished in the next few hours, days, weeks, or months, and long-range goals, which may take years to accomplish. Your list may look something like this:

- begin an exercise program
- write an article for publication
- join the tennis club
- volunteer for Red Cross work
- complete my baccalaureate in nursing
- become certified as a critical care nurse

Writing your goals down helps you commit yourself to their attainment. Your next step is to prioritize your goals. This may be a bit more difficult than generating goals, but it will help you to resolve any conflict you may have about which goal to pursue. Setting priorities also helps you focus your time based on which of your goals is most important. The rank order of your goals may look like this:

1. begin an exercise program
2. complete my baccalaureate in nursing
3. become certified as a critical care nurse
4. volunteer for Red Cross work
5. join the tennis club
6. write an article for publication

In this example, your personal goal of beginning an exercise program is your top priority, and should not interfere with your simultaneous attainment of other goals. In another instance, you may find you have first to achieve the goal listed as top priority before you can attempt to meet the other goals listed.

Once your goals are listed in order of priority, you can then plan strategies to help you achieve them. This is useful particularly with long-range goals that will require more time and energy expenditure than short-range goals.

Include for each of your goals a target date for completion. Setting a date by which the specific goal should have been achieved will provide motivation for you and reinforcement for your efforts when the goal is attained. A periodic review of your goals and your progress toward attaining them also will help keep you "on target."

Now that you have some idea of your professional goals, some immediate and some rather long range, the next step is assessing your current situation to see how well your goals can be achieved by staying where you are. Networking has a special characteristic in that it can be helpful in both situations—the one where you decide you like where you are and will stay there, and the one where you decide it's time to move up and out! Networking can help nurses at all stages of their nursing career and at all levels in the profession.

ILLUSTRATIONS OF ACHIEVING GOALS

To illustrate a situation in which a nurse's present position offers her the career advancement she wants, let's get acquainted with Sally Roberts. Sally is a baccalaureate graduate with three years experience in intensive care nursing. Sally works in a large medical center hospital; she is currently on the afternoon shift. She is not married, but is going steady with prospects for an engagement in the near future. Sally has been taking classes at the local university for the past several semesters, "halfheartedly" working on a master's degree in nursing service administration.

Sally has not had a position in nursing beyond that of night charge nurse. There is, however, a day shift position opening soon with the resignation of the assistant head nurse. The assistant head nurse who is resigning was a college classmate and she told Sally several weeks ago that she was leaving. Sally is very much interested in that position. She would like to try working in such an administrative position before she goes much further with her graduate study in nursing administration. She is committed to a career in nursing and has set as her ultimate goal to become the vice president for nursing at a medical center hospital. Her concern about moving into an administrative position is based on not knowing whether she would be a good supervisor and whether she would regret leaving the clinical aspect of nursing practice.

Notice about the availability of the position has not yet been posted, but a public announcement is imminent. Sally's boyfriend is encouraging her to apply for the position before the vacancy is announced, "to get the jump on it." Sally is uncertain about the advisability of the approach, but she wants the position. The methods that Sally would use to achieve her goal (obtaining the position as assistant head nurse of the intensive care unit) are somewhat different from those that would be used by a nurse for whom there are not career advancement opportunities in her present employment setting.

This nurse is Anne Gorden, on the faculty in a school of nursing. Anne is exceptionally well prepared to teach psychiatric/mental health nursing to graduate students. She has a master's degree in nursing with a clinical specialty in psychiatric nursing. She is almost finished with a doctorate (ABD—all but dissertation) in clinical psychology (with an emphasis on child growth and development). Anne is married and the mother of two school-age children. Her husband is also on the faculty of the university, in the English Department. Anne has not yet been tenured at the university; eligibility criteria for tenure have been tightened recently because of the large number of tenured faculty and the declining student enrollment. Anne has been in the same position for five years. "It's time for a change," she sighs, "but my husband won't leave here, so I'm stuck, too."

Anne's professional goals have been carefully and specifically defined. She wants to establish herself in the field as an expert in stepparenting, an area she feels has not yet been fully explored by any of the professions dealing with emotional problems of people. Anne feels strongly that she must move to an urban area where there are more varied opportunities for professional growth and career advancement in order to achieve her major professional goal. Anne hasn't talked with anyone about her aspirations because "it wouldn't do any good." Several of her closest friends are aware of Anne's increasing frustration, but attribute it to her hectic schedule encompassing work, home, and school.

The individuals in both of these illustrations have set their professional goals. Both know where they want to go in their careers, but will need to use somewhat different methods to get there. In both instances, however, networking skills can help them.

Both need to carefully assess their current situations and use their existing networks to get what they want. In both cases, information is essential. Sally needs to know more about the position of assistant head nurse: when the position vacancy will be announced, who else might be a candidate for the position, what the person making the selection for the position thinks about her candidacy, and so on. Anne needs to know about other avenues for achieving her goal besides moving to another location. Both can benefit from feedback from others in their network: Are their expectations realistic? Do they have the potential to accomplish what they want to? Are the strategies they've selected to get what they want appropriate? Will they work? And so on.

Both nurses can benefit from another advantage of networking, which is referral. Sally needs a specific referral for a specific situation. Anne will benefit more from general referrals in several situations. A referral to the person making the decision about the assistant head nurse position from someone in a position of influence could well be a key factor in Sally's getting the position. For example, the present assistant head nurse (the incumbent) says, "I understand that Sally Roberts is interested in my position when I leave. I've always been impressed with Sally's clinical skills. She's now working on her master's in nursing service administration, which shows that she's serious about wanting to learn more and grow professionally. Even though she's relatively new here, she has demonstrated leadership ability; she organized the patient care conferences, which are such a success.

It's obvious to me that she gives considerable thought to the performance appraisals for the staff on her shift; they're among the best ones done on this unit. I've noticed better working relationships among the nurses on night shift since she's been in charge. I think she's ready to move into a position with more responsibility. What do you think about her taking the assistant head nurse position when I resign?"

Anne, too, can benefit from being referred to others. There may be an individual in the community where Anne lives who also is interested in the topic of stepparenting and who can be of help to Anne. If her interest in the topic is known to others, they can serve as her "agents" when the opportunity arises.

For example, a nurse who is on the faculty with Anne is also on the program committee for the local mental health association. During the committee meeting, when the group is planning educational sessions for the remainder of the year, the nurse says, "I've noticed that the Crisis Center Hot-Line has received an increasing number of telephone calls from stepparents and stepchildren lately. With the divorce rate rising as high as it has been, it's no wonder that there are so many second families occurring. It's got to be a difficult situation from both sides. I wonder if it wouldn't be appropriate for us to present some sort of workshop for the general public on that topic? As a matter of fact, one of the faculty members I work with, Anne Gorden, has some expertise on the topic. I'm sure she would be willing to teach; would you like me to ask her?"

Thus, Anne's exposure to the community as an "expert" on stepparenting is initiated. Assuming she does a good job at the workshop, there could be additional contacts made with offers for more teaching opportunities, consultation, and so on.

Besides these two brief examples, there are many other methods Sally and Anne could use that would assist them in attaining their professional career goals. All of these strategies are integral components of the networking process that will contribute to your professional growth. Presenting yourself well as you network involves other strategies that also can contribute to your professional growth, including:

- speaking effectively in public
- being assertive
- making changes
- using your power

PUBLIC SPEAKING

Public speaking causes great difficulty for many people. Women, particularly, have been "taught to form habits of word use . . . that directly contradict the purpose of communication: exchanging ideas and sharing feelings," according to the authors of the book *Speaking Up*.[2] Women have been convinced from their early years that the assets of a good speaker, such as a strong voice, direct eye contact, self-confidence, good posture, and clear-cut, decisive speech aren't "feminine." Nurses, however, are continuously in professional roles in which they must speak up and speak effectively.

There are techniques that can be applied by nurses who want to increase or improve their public speaking ability, whether in giving a speech from a platform, discussing a patient's care with the physician, describing a care plan to a group of peers, or being interviewed for a new job.[3] In this context, all speaking is public speaking, and nurses must prepare themselves to do it well.

A most helpful technique in learning to speak well in public is to listen to yourself, using a cassette recorder, or to listen and watch yourself, using a videotape recorder, as you give a speech. In this way you can get feedback about your public speaking ability.

Even if you don't have access to videotaping equipment, most of us do have access to an audio cassette tape recorder, so, at the minimum, you can hear yourself talk. Continuing education classes on public speaking or communication skills may use video equipment; such classes are relatively inexpensive and well worth the financial and time investment. (Contact your local university continuing education department to see if such classes are available in your area.)

If you don't have access to such recording equipment, you should get feedback about your speaking from others, such as your friends, network, or family members. A group organized to promote good public speaking is the Toastmasters International. (There are chapters in almost every urban area; check the phone book for a listing.) This group meets frequently, usually in a social environment such as a restaurant. The members practice public speaking, giving each other useful feedback. Members of Toastmasters are heavily in demand as banquet speakers, which gives testimony to the group's success. While the speeches given by members of this group are not generally similar to the "professional" speeches nurses would be making, the principles of good public speaking learned through association with the Toastmasters can be applied to all situations in which nurses and others must speak in front of an audience of any size.

When you record yourself, try to do it in as many situations as possible, both professional and personal. Taping only carefully prepared and delivered professional talks may not let you hear what you sound like when you laugh in a more spontaneous situation. When you have numerous recordings listen to them and try to analyze your speaking voice.

Listen carefully for the pitch of your voice. If it is too high, so that you sound like a small child, you may want to practice lowering it, taping your efforts and listening to find a pitch you find more pleasing, then concentrating your continued practice on that pitch. The pitch of your voice can be lowered with practice. Listening to recordings of your voice when you are amused or angry will convince you that the pitch of your voice already does change. You need only to convince yourself that you can practice changing it at will.

If your voice sounds nasal, it may be because you are feeling tense as you are speaking. Listen to tape recordings of your voice in more relaxed situations to see if there is a difference. A nasal tone generally is associated with a complaint so listen to the content of the message. You can practice reducing the nasal tone in your voice by consciously trying to eliminate it and listening to find which of your efforts produces a tone that sounds better to you.

The volume of your voice is another aspect you should listen for. If you talk softly, so that you barely can be heard, you will not command much attention when you speak. A strong voice, not a weak one, is an asset for an effective speaker. Practice raising your voice and listening to it. In this instance, however, you may need to rely on others' feedback about the best volume, since they would be in the audience when you speak and would need to hear you clearly.

If you have access to a videotape of you speaking, you will be able to assess not only your voice, but your behavior while talking. If not, practice talking in front of a mirror, or in front of friends who will give you feedback on how you look as you talk.

If you're in front of a mirror, observe carefully how you stand as you talk. Do you slouch, cross your arms in front of you, or grip the podium so tightly that your knuckles are white? Do you play with your hair, your pen, your clothes, the light on the podium? In all of these instances, you appear less than relaxed and self-confident about your speaking, and this attitude is quickly communicated to your audience.

Pay attention to other aspects of your delivery of a speech. For example, do you talk too fast or too slowly? Are you afflicted with a "nervous giggle" when you're not saying anything humorous? Are you smiling inappropriately? What does your facial expression say? Where are you looking, at the ceiling, the floor, or the wall at the back of the room?

Ask your friends to tell you the two or three things they liked about the way you looked or sounded as you spoke and the two or three things they didn't like. Listen carefully, and undefensively, to make the most of what is constructive in what they say. At Toastmasters such critiques are a necessary component of every speech, whether rehearsed or spontaneous.

Common Poor Speech Habits

As important as how you look and how your voice sounds when you speak is what you say. Women often possess many negative speaking habits of which they may be completely unaware. Listening to yourself speak in a variety of situations may make those speech patterns more apparent to you so that you may begin to correct them. Among the most common are:

- nervous mannerisms
- insecurity
- jargon
- pomposity

The worst offender to the listener's ear is nervous mannerisms of speech, such as the "ums," "ers," and "I means." Weed these noises out of your speech, whether you are speaking from a prepared text or on the spur of the moment. Another gross offender is the tag "you know?" at the end of each sentence you say. Feedback from your tapes and/or your friends combined with conscientious practice will eliminate these barriers to effective speaking.

Insecurity in speaking manifests itself in many ways, of which the most obvious is qualifying every statement. Typical qualifiers include "If you

don't mind my saying it, I think. . . ., " "I'd sort of like to tell you. . . .,"
"If I could say something about that. . . ., " and so on.

Reinforcing statements with words of emphasis is another example of
insecure speech patterns. Examples include such statements as "It was
really terrible. . . ., " "I'm really not certain about. . . ., " "I just think
we should. . . ., " and "I just don't know what to do. . . ."

Self-effacement is another negative speech pattern particularly common
to women. Often nurses don't assert their true opinions without modifying
them in some manner, such as "I suppose that new medication is causing
some of Mr. Ball's loss of appetite," "I'm going to assign you to Mrs.
Geovanni today, ok?" or "I guess we ought to start on the performance
appraisals, don't you think?"

In contrast, men's speech is characterized by the absence of such self-
effacement. A man typically would say "Loss of appetite is a side effect
of that medication; that explains Mr. Ball's decreased food intake," "You
have Mrs. Geovanni today," and "It's time to start on the performance
appraisals."

Astutely listening to conversations in which both men and women participate will increase your awareness of the negative and positive speaking
patterns of both sexes. This information can be used to your advantage in
your future communications with either sex.

Jargon also is offensive to the listener. One of the most frequent forms
of jargon is the use of acronyms. While most acronyms you use may be
familiar to your audience, many are not and your listeners will find it
frustrating to listen to you. If you use acronyms, explain their meaning
the first time you use them. For example, you may say "A common nursing
intervention in Disseminated Intervascular Coagulation, or DIC for short,
is. . . ., " or "The incidence of Adult Respiratory Distress Syndrome,
also known as ARDS, has increased over the last decade. . . . "

Another form of jargon is the use of "faddish" words or phrases, such
as "I would like to share with you. . . .," "We shared that information.
. . ., " or "They will be sharing the results of the study. . . . " Another
recent offender is the use of the word "impact" as a verb (although some
recently published dictionaries, perhaps in concession to common use,
are listing as a variant of the noun impact the verb form), as in "The
decreased staffing is impacting on the quality of patient care," or "I
anticipate that the change will impact on our unit more than on most."
Frequent use of such phrases can detract from the content of what you
are saying.

Pompous language is insulting to the audience, particularly when pref-
aced with "For those of you who don't know. . . ., " or "If you are not
familiar with the word, it means. . . ., " and so on. If a word has to be

explained to the audience, another word probably would be better in its place. If no other word will do, then define the word clearly without prefacing remarks.

If you don't use the word in your everyday speaking, then don't use it in a prepared speech. Use of "twenty-five cent" words often is thought to indicate the sophistication or scholarliness of the speaker, but the effect generally is the opposite; the speaker appears to be trying to impress the listeners.

Practice will help you improve your public speaking ability. When you've mastered those aspects of your public speaking ability on which you chose to focus your efforts, you are ready to move on to conquer your fear of speaking in public.

Fear of Public Speaking

Others, in addition to nurses, experience the sweaty palms and butter-flies in the stomach that precede making a speech from the podium. Fear of public speaking is quite common, but it can be overcome, say Stone and Bachner, authors of *Speaking Up.*[4]

There are ways that have been proven effective in limiting anxiety about speaking in public. Many fledgling public speakers are given such (unhelp-ful) advice as "Imagine all of the people in the audience are in their underwear and how ridiculous they look, and you won't be nervous" or "They all put on their pants the same way you do, one leg at a time, so they're no different; nothing to worry about!"

Perhaps more helpful is the knowledge that a bit of anxiety helps an individual do better. The key is to keep the anxiety at a manageable level, so that it doesn't escalate into panic. A short-term strategy is to recognize that the danger of giving a public speech is not physical; you will come to no harm if you don't do well. The speech will be given and it will be over. You can nurse your wounds in private if you think you haven't done as well as you would have liked (and often we are harder on ourselves with criticism than others might be).

A more long-term strategy for handling the fear of public speaking is to realize that the fear lessens with practice. The more you speak in public, the less uncomfortable it will become. In fact, although this may be hard to believe, the first time you speak to an audience and your customary prespeech jitters aren't there, you will miss the tingle of excitement you'd previously had!

The best overall strategy is to recognize that you will improve over time. Each time will be better than the last, if you constantly strive to improve your public speaking ability. You have to start somewhere, and the somewhere you are starting may be at the very beginning, but you won't be there long. Each time you speak you will be further from your starting point than you were the time before.

Using your experiences to help you progress is essential. You may progress slowly and painfully or easily and rapidly, but, either way, you will progress. You have to practice in order to speak well; you can practice by yourself, in front of friends, in a class on public speaking, as a member of Toastmasters, and at every opportunity, but the most important thing is that you practice!

Being nervous can cause us to make mistakes we wouldn't ordinarily make. These mistakes may seem trivial in private, but in front of an audience they assume mountainous proportions. You may just have been introduced and find you can't start your speech. The length of time that elapses between the end of your introduction and the start of your speech will seem much longer to you than to the audience. When you make this mistake or any other you must realize that you can continue, appearing not to have made a mistake, or you can get more anxious and upset and compound what is, up to this point, a very minor mistake, if a mistake at all.

One helpful technique in preparing for a speech before an audience is to think about all the mistakes you possibly could make and plan strategies to overcome them. All of the mistakes you think about couldn't possibly happen to you, even in an entire career of public speaking, but this will tend to minimize the terror of "what if?"

Most public speakers have fears that fall into several major categories. Among these are:

- forgetting what to say
- getting physically ill
- saying the wrong thing
- being clumsy
- boring the audience

Forgetting What To Say

One fairly common fear, caused by anxiety, is that you will forget what you want to say. Again, the time lapse that occurs between when you go blank and when you pick up the train of your thought will appear longer to you than to your audience. It is important to remain calm, so that the anxiety you are experiencing isn't communicated to the audience. Try hard not to stutter and stammer as you look for the word you need, or find your place in your notes or outline.

Adequate preparation for your speech, in the form of notes or an outline and lots of practice in delivering your speech, will assist you to overcome this fear. Don't be afraid to refer to your notes, reading them if necessary to get you past your temporary lapse. When you feel more comfortable you can begin again to talk without relying as much on your notes.

Getting Sick

Getting physically ill can be the result of excessive anxiety. You already should know how your body responds to anxiety and so can prepare for similar response when you are going to give a public speech. If you tend to be nauseated, avoid eating before your speech. If you generally have diarrhea, avoid eating before your talk, and know where the bathrooms are. You may wish to take an antispasmodic or mild tranquilizer before you give your talk, but it's not wise to rely on such chemical crutches on a long-term basis.

Similarly, avoid having a drink or two "to relax" before giving an after-dinner speech, even if there is a cocktail hour before the dinner. With a high anxiety level, alcohol will be more likely to impair your speech and coordination, perhaps with disastrous effect.

Other Physical Effects

The physical effects of your anxiety may manifest themselves in less dramatic ways. You simply may experience sweaty palms, underarms, or a dry mouth. There is little to be done about excessive perspiration due to anxiety. Carry a cloth handkerchief with which to inconspicuously dry your hands. A paper tissue won't do in this event; it will quickly get soggy and be utterly useless.

You may wish to use dress shields to avoid staining your expensive clothes. Applying a good antiperspirant to your underarms when you shower or bathe should relieve your worries about perspiration odor. If you are concerned about having perspiration odor when you mingle with the audience after you've given a talk, wear a dress with a jacket. Remove the jacket during your speech and put it on again before you join the audience. Even if you've perspired a lot during your talk, with the jacket on as a cover-up, you won't need to worry about perspiration odor.

If your mouth is dry you will want to have water at the podium. If water hasn't been provided, then ask for it. You will appear self-confident and relaxed as you sip water casually during your talk. Remember that the time you use to take a sip of water again seems longer to you than to the audience. Avoid huge gulps of water, particularly if you are very tense; you don't want to choke, cough, or splutter.

Some people chew gum or candy as they give a speech, but choking or swallowing wrong can be a problem. Drinking water in small sips, just enough to wet the mouth each time, is more effective. Applying chapstick before giving a talk will help keep the lips moist.

Saying the Wrong Thing

Public speakers often worry about saying the wrong thing. If you've prepared well and practiced your speech you should already have eliminated offensive material, such as sexist language (he and his, or when addressing nurses, she and hers), or stereotypical references such as to foreigners, physicians, or ethnic groups. You will have cleansed your speech of obscene language or inappropriate humor. Nothing in the planned content, then, should cause concern.

What does cause concern, and some anticipatory anxiety, is what you may say spontaneously. You may be reassured to know that everyone makes such a mistake at one time or another. The audience reaction is quite often laughter, because the mistake is a humorous one. They are not laughing at you but at the humor in what you said, or, rather, mis-said.

If you can laugh at the mistake yourself, you will appear more self-confident and relaxed than if you apologize profusely and attempt to correct the mistake. If you can't laugh along with the audience, remain quiet until the laughter has died before you resume. Correct the mistake and move on. Even if you miss a section of your talk, your correction should be made calmly and matter-of-factly. Profuse apologies or agonizing aloud over a mistake makes the audience uncomfortable for themselves and for you.

Being Clumsy

All of the above problems pale in comparison with being clumsy. What if you trip over the microphone cord or, as you're writing on it, the flip chart falls, or, worse yet, you fall? Those are instances of which nightmares are made. Fortunately, such extreme instances of ungainliness don't occur often.

One way to combat the fear that they might happen to you is to prepare for such eventualities. If you have access to the room in advance of the time when you are giving your speech, practice walking to the podium from your seat. Check on the electrical cords for audiovisual equipment, lights, and the microphone. If they are lying loose on the floor in your path, ask to have them taped down. Check on the sturdiness of the equipment carts, the flip chart, the slateboard, if portable, and so on.

The time to fix accidents is before they happen. You can take precautions to avoid accidents; don't wear new leather-soled shoes without "scuffing" them on concrete first so they won't slip. Don't wear your highest heels or wedges on a platform stage. Avoid wearing bracelets that can get caught on the edge of the podium.

If an accident does occur, the audience generally will respond with laughter. Unlike when you make a mistake, this laugh is not in response to something humorous; the audience is uncomfortable for you. You will only increase their discomfort if you respond to the accident by being uncomfortable yourself. As difficult as it may be, handle the situation with composure, and even humor, if you can manage it. The humor shouldn't be self-deprecating: "I sure am clumsy today." Such humor only increases the audience's discomfort and does nothing to remedy the situation.

Planning for such disasters can greatly mitigate their effects. Rehearsing your recovery plans on your friends can provide you with feedback on the most effective responses from an audience's perspective to mistakes you may make.

Boring the Audience

The final disaster, from which there may be no recovery, is boring your audience. Activities engaged in by people who are bored include reading (something other than your handouts), talking to the person sitting in the next seat, yawning, fidgeting in the seat, and worst of all, sleeping. Almost every audience, bar none, contains a few individuals who will be doing something besides listening during your talk.

It is important that you assess what is going on if a large part of your audience is bored. If you have talked long past your allotted time, fidgeting people are a clue that it is time to stop. Yawning and other signs of boredom may simply be because you are giving an after-dinner speech to people sated with food and drink who are, as a result, naturally tired. Individuals in an audience who are sleeping may be doing so because it is the middle of the day; they work nights and this is their usual time to sleep.

The problem may be with your delivery. If you are giving your talk in a monotone or in a low voice, with little variation in your tone, then you may be the cause of the boredom. Try to put more enthusiasm in your speech. If your content is too basic or too advanced for your audience, they will be inattentive. Knowing in advance the composition of your audience will help eliminate this problem.

If you determine that the problem is not your fault, but that of those in the audience who are bored, focus your attention on individuals who are not bored. Find someone who is interested and attentive, and deliver the remainder of your speech to that person. The positive reinforcement will be helpful to you as you proceed.

If you sense that the audience is tired, you may wish to cut short the talk and ask for questions. People may be less bored when they have the opportunity to interact with you. Keep your responses to questions brief, so that you won't get back into a "lecture" format. If there are no questions, pose one or two yourself, such as "I usually get asked whether there are any advantages to the method I've proposed. The major advantage I see is. . . . " Again, the response to your self-generated question should be brief. This tactic may spark some questions from members of the audience. If not, it's better to close gracefully without apology. At the very least you've had another opportunity to practice your public speaking skills, and you've learned something from it which should allow you to improve for the next time.

BEING ASSERTIVE

Women in the health care system, as in society in general, have been the silent majority. Although they outnumber men, rarely have women had much of a say in the policies that govern their lives. Many of us blame men for this situation; after all, they control the system and it's the system that oppresses us. Elizabeth Janeway, noted sociologist and author of *Man's World, Woman's Place,* says, "If there's nothing more powerful than an idea whose time has come, there is nothing more ubiquitously pervasive than an idea whose time won't go."[5] An idea whose time must go is that women are powerless to do anything about the system in which they live and work. Women can, and do, make a difference. One means through which nurses are discovering that they can make a difference is by becoming assertive.

Women have a long history of being nonassertive individuals and nurses are no different from women in general. Being nonassertive has not helped nurses as individuals or nursing as a profession. Learning to be assertive has offered nurses the opportunity to practice techniques that will help them set their own goals and attain them.

Learning to be assertive is an integral component of networking. If you're not assertive you won't speak up about yourself or what you want. You probably won't get help from those who can help you to get what you want if you don't take the initiative to seek them out and enlist their support.

Self-respect and self-esteem are basic to the ability to be assertive. In order to be effectively assertive, you must be pleased with who you are and where you are going. In the section on values clarification you learned how to identify your personal and professional goals. Assertiveness is one strategy you can use to help achieve those goals that you identified as important.

There are numerous techniques you can practice to initiate or improve your assertive behavior. Among the most useful are:

- expressing your thoughts directly
- using assertive language

When you express your thoughts directly you use statements that generally begin with "I," such as "I think," "I feel," or "I believe." You stand up for what you think, feel, or believe in a way that indicates that you assume responsibility for those thoughts, feelings, and beliefs. In contrast, a nonassertive response is "You make me feel," "You think that I," or "You seem to believe that I." Practice in using direct statements of your thoughts will ultimately make it easier for you to say "I want" or "I need."

Direct statements to individuals are more assertive than similar statements to a group. For example, the head nurse who says "We all know that the narcotic keys are the responsibility of the medication nurse" is less assertive (and less effective) than when she says to the offending nurse "Miss Ayres, you are aware that it is the medication nurse's responsibility to keep the narcotic keys." Other examples of indirect and, consequently, nonassertive statements include "You can't expect that we. . . .," "It is generally true that . . . .," "It seems to us that . . . .," and "As you well know. . . ."

Using assertive language is an important assertiveness technique. Telling someone that you won't do something implies that you are more in control of yourself and what you will do than when you tell someone you can't do something. When you use assertive language, your statement might sound like this: "You said you would have the report ready by today, but you haven't turned it in yet." A nonassertive statement in the same instance might sound like: "Gosh, isn't this the day the reports are due?" Assertive techniques are more effective than hinting, or, worse yet, being angry but not communicating that feeling to the person with whom you are angry.

Nurses' Rights

Another way of viewing assertiveness is as a strategy to help you attain your rights as a woman in the health professions, as identified by Melodie

Chenevert, formerly Instructor, University of Wisconsin, School of Nursing, Madison, and author of *Special Techniques in Assertiveness Training for Women in the Health Professions.*[6] Chenevert lists, among these, the right to:

- be treated with respect
- have a reasonable workload
- be paid a just wage
- determine your own priorities
- ask for what you want (or need)
- say "no" without feeling guilty
- make mistakes
- be accountable for your actions
- exchange information on a professional basis
- act in the best interest of your patients/clients
- be a human being

In order to expect respect from others, we first must respect ourselves. If we respect ourselves, it will be easier to speak up in instances when others don't respect us. Note this example of an instance where an occupational health nurse is told to assume responsibilities that are clearly not related to the nursing role. The nurse responds to the Personnel Officer, "I really understand that it puts you in a bind when the switchboard operator doesn't come to work until 7 A.M. and workers call in starting at 6 A.M., but I have most of my charting and filing to do between 6 A.M. and 7 A.M. In addition, I find that [night shift] employees often come to see me right before going home at 7 A.M. To take on the additional task of call-ins would overload me. I cannot do it at this time."[7] Here the nurse's assertive response reflects respect for his or her professional role and responsibility, which he or she feels and which the Personnel Office also must feel.

Nurses have a right not to be overworked. In this era of nurse shortages, nurses often are made to feel guilty if they don't accomplish all that they are assigned during their workday. In some situations, nurses experience "burn-out" as a result of overwork; in others, nurses simply leave the profession in order to escape unreasonable demands. Assertiveness will help the nurse in such a situation to make demands about a reasonable workload. Nurses trying to make such changes in their work situations would do well to plan effective change strategies. Often, nurses working together in an organized manner are able to accomplish much more than a nurse working alone to change the system.

Equitable pay for nurses is an issue that has received much attention recently. Again, nurses working together may be able to accomplish more in relation to improved salaries than one nurse alone.

Nurses have the right to determine their own priorities. This should be as true in your personal life as in your professional life. Once you've identified your goals you should attempt to achieve them. Often this entails delegating responsibility for tasks that were thought of as your "job" but that you can't do if you are to achieve the goals most important to you. An illustration is when you are assertive with your husband in expecting him to share in household responsibilities so that you can attend evening classes at the local college to complete your baccalaureate in nursing. Or when you delegate some routine paperwork to the ward clerk so that you can spend some extra time in providing emotional support to a patient about to undergo surgery for a suspected malignancy.

Nurses have the right to ask for what they want and what they need. Many nurses are able to quickly list items that would help them improve their patient care, but are reluctant to request that they receive them. Often the response to a request, when it is finally made, is positive. An assertive request for what is needed should be made in a calm, rational manner, such as in this example: "The rate of hypertension among workers in this industry is quite high. It is difficult to monitor these employees' progress without frequent blood pressure checks. The accuracy of blood pressure measurement is doubtful if the appropriate size cuff is not used. I need several sizes of blood pressure cuffs for the employees I am currently following. Here is a list of the sizes I need; when will you order them?"

It is extremely difficult for nurses to say "no." Nurses need to realize that not saying no to someone else when they wish to is, in effect, saying no to themselves. As with many other assertive techniques, saying no gets easier with practice. Saying no also is easier if the nurse recognizes as basic his or her right to be treated with respect and to be assigned a reasonable workload. A most awkward position for many nurses is saying no to a physician. In instances where nurses are concerned about a physician's order for medications that may be either in the wrong dose or in a dangerous combination with another drug, the nurse must be guided by the right to act on behalf of the patient/client as well as his or her legal responsibility.

Nurses have the right to make mistakes. When infractions are minor, they should be treated as such. For example, the nurse who makes minor errors in records or reports should be cautioned about not continuing to do so, but there is no need to "make a federal case out of it," as often happens.

Many nurses are reluctant to speak up for their rights for fear of being "wrong," particularly in instances where in the past being "wrong" has been a painful experience. Consider, for example, a nurse who thinks assessing pupil response is within the responsibilities of a nurse when assessing a patient (and rightly so!). The nurse is reported to nursing administration by a physician who feels it is a medical not a nursing responsibility. In deference to the physician's wishes, the nurse is told to discontinue the practice of checking pupil response. That nurse will not be very likely to practice nursing assessment in the future, nor defend the right and obligation of nurses to check pupil responses of their patients.

Nurses have the right to give and receive information on a professional basis. That is, they have a right to know the patient's medical care plan from the physician. They have a right to talk with the patient and family about the care plan. Nurses who abdicate this right are not meeting their professional responsibilities. Assertive responses are useful here in helping others see that you are aware of and intend to exercise your rights. For example, the nurse says to the attending physician: "Dr. Collins, Mrs. Margot is quite concerned about the possibility of having a mastectomy. She brought with her to the hospital an article that appeared in a recent issue of a women's magazine. We have just discussed the alternatives to a radical mastectomy described in the article. We wrote down together some more specific questions about some of those alternatives, which she will be asking you. Her husband wishes to be there when you talk with her. When can I tell them it will be convenient for you to meet with them?"

Finally, nurses have the right to be human beings. They have the right to be angry or frustrated in a work situation with which they cannot cope. They have the right to go into the linen closet and scream into a stack of pillowcases when a physician has been rude. They have the right to cry when a supervisor unjustly berates them in front of others. Nurses have the right to laugh, to love, and to be happy.

Along with these rights, nurses must be accountable for their own actions. It is a professional's duty to be responsible for his or her own actions. Thus, nurses are responsible for not taking action in situations where some action is necessary and justified.

Being assertive is one way to help assure yourself that you can have all of these rights and others. At the same time, being assertive will help you be a professional nurse who is fully meeting his or her responsibilities as well.

Assertiveness Guidelines

General guidelines for becoming assertive include:

- start with a situation that will result in a success

- learn to be persistent
- avoid getting angry
- practice saying "no"
- use positive communication

It's wise to practice being assertive in a situation where you don't have a lot to lose. If your first try results in not succeeding you will be less inclined to try again. Trying an assertive technique with a family member for the first time is difficult, something you need to work up to. Start with a telephone solicitor instead, for example, one who begins the sales pitch by saying he is a handicapped worker who makes his livelihood by selling kitchen brooms. If you've previously responded to such ploys you will feel a sense of accomplishment when you simply say "No, thank you, I'm not interested."

Next try being assertive in a person-to-person situation, such as when you've waited in line for some time and the clerk offers to wait on the woman next to you. You calmly say, without apology, "I'm next; I would like to see the black leather gloves, please, in size 7." Once you've practiced a bit in situations where success is highly likely, you'll be ready to try assertiveness techniques with your family members and at work.

Being persistent is important in assertiveness. Often a nurse will make a request, and when it is turned down, the nurse may think the denial unfair but rarely does anything else about it. In being assertive you must learn to pursue your objective. Here the "broken record" technique will be useful. This technique involves repetition of your original response, varying the way the response is worded, but not providing additional "fuel for the fire." An example that contrasts a nonassertive response with an assertive, "broken record," response follows.

Martha has been asked to take call for the operating room during the night shift. It is the third time this week she has taken call. She and her husband planned to go out for dinner with friends this evening. It will be a late evening and she does not wish to be on call during the night. The supervisor waits for Martha's answer.

> *Martha:* Why don't you ask Susan instead of me?
> *Supervisor:* You know why; you're a better O.R. nurse. Besides, if I went around asking everybody you suggest I'd get nothing else done today.
> *Martha:* I've done it three times already!
> *Supervisor:* Somebody has to do it; you know we can't leave the O.R. uncovered.

Martha: (annoyed): I'm tired; I need my sleep.
Supervisor: You won't get called anyway; it's been quiet lately.
Martha: (resigned): Well, all right, but this is the last time, you hear?

Consider now Martha's changed approach to the supervisor's request:

Martha: I'm sorry; I'm just not able to take call tonight.
Supervisor: Do you have plans tonight?
Martha: Yes, and so it's not convenient for me to take call.
Supervisor: Who will I get if you don't do it?
Martha: I don't know; I'm unable to do it.
Supervisor: Are you sure you can't? I'm in a terrible bind.
Martha: I'm sure.
Supervisor: Well I'll just have to find someone else if you won't; the O.R. has to be covered. Can you think of someone I can ask?
Martha: I'm sorry, I can't suggest anyone.
Supervisor: Never mind, I'll find someone.

With the latter exchange, Martha said the same thing in several ways. She was a "broken record," repeating the same message using different words until the supervisor understood clearly what Martha was trying to convey.

An important part of effectively using assertive responses is not getting angry or annoyed. Stating what you think and feel in a calm, purposeful manner is essential. Avoid getting into an argument with the other person. Arguing will quickly defeat your purpose. Use the broken record technique instead of involving yourself in a circular discussion. Listen carefully to the other person and respond to his or her feelings about the situations: "I can understand that you are frustrated, upset, angry, disappointed, etc., but. . . ."

Again, practice will help you perfect your techniques for saying no. Start small, in situations where it won't matter much if you end up saying yes instead. Any practice you get ultimately will help you say no in a situation where it will mean a lot to you. You can say "no" or "no, thank you," but the important word to convey is no. Here are examples of capably saying no:

Nurse, asked to assume a committee assignment in addition to her other responsibilities, says "No, thank you, but I can't accept an assignment to that committee at this time."

Nurse, being asked to take care of an additional patient because another nurse wants to leave work early, says "I'm sorry, but I can't take on the responsibility of another patient and give adequate care to those I'm already assigned.''

In both these instances the nurse did not accept additional work, refusing calmly. In both instances, if persistence was necessary, the nurse could have rephrased her response but still said no, without offering excuses for refusing, or feeling guilty and ending up by saying yes.

When you use assertive responses, couch them in positive rather than negative terms. If you ask a question in a manner that suggests that you expect a negative answer, such as "You don't want to order these extra supplies, do you?" you will most likely get exactly that "no" response. Statements such as "I suppose you don't want to go over the assignment sheet right now" and "I imagine we're too short staffed all over to get some extra help for this unit" also will be likely to elicit a negative response.

Avoid minimizing your request, as in "This is not very important, but . . . . " or "I know you're busy right now and I hate to bother you, but . . . . " A positive statement or question will imply to the listener that you expect a positive response.

Assertiveness is one way for nurses to make changes in the systems in which they live and work. Because there are many changes to be made, an organized, effective approach is needed. Such an approach is now available through the body of knowledge about change.

MAKING CHANGES

Nurses have understood for years the need to make changes in the health care system. All of the frustrations of the system and the profession are illustrated by the occupational health nurse who says "They won't let us make changes around here." Some of the reason the change didn't occur becomes apparent when the nurse next says "I've been complaining about that situation ever since I first started working here, but nobody listens. Pretty soon I just quit talking about it. Nothing does any good. They won't change." Or, take the case of the staff nurse who says about an aide who won't carry her share of the workload, "Yeah, I told the head nurse and the supervisor about her, but nothing happened. It doesn't do any good to try to change things in this place."

In each of these instances, how the two nurses who wanted to make changes approached the desired change had an influence on the probability that the change actually would happen. In order to make changes happen, nurses have to know about the change process. A useful text specifically for nurses about the change process has been written by Ingeborg G.

Mauksch, Professor of Nursing, School of Nursing, Vanderbilt University, and Michael H. Miller, a sociologist and Associate Professor of Nursing in the School of Nursing at Vanderbilt University. It is titled *Implementing Change in Nursing*.

In their book, Mauksch and Miller describe change as an alteration in an individual or a system.[8] The person who is instrumental in planning for an alteration in the system is a change agent. The change agent acts deliberately and systematically to assess the system and analyze all aspects of the situation within the system that must be changed. To accomplish the change, the nurse change agent must have a perspective of the system, the problem, and the potential solution to the problem that requires change.

Change can be either planned or unplanned. Most unplanned change occurs through the efforts of those who work in opposition to the existing authority structure in the system. New nursing graduates often are responsible for unplanned change as they oppose the status quo, the "we've always done it this way" syndrome. Nurses who attend continuing education activities and bring back new ideas they've learned and suggest new methods to be tried also are responsible for much of the unplanned change that occurs in health care settings.

Unfortunately, such spontaneous occurrences may reflect poorly on the nurses who were the cause of the change. Typically these nurses are labeled "troublemakers" and are accused of "trying to make waves." Some nurses leave the profession as a result of being harassed because they are trying to change things; other nurses respond by "not trying anymore—what's the use?"

Planned change, in contrast to unplanned change, is organized, systematic, and generally more effective. Planned change doesn't adversely affect the change agent. The outcome of planned change is usually positive; whereas the outcome of unplanned change varies.

How To Plan Change

In order to effectively plan and implement change, nurses must: (1) understand a theory of change and (2) have the characteristics of a change agent. Systems theory is perhaps the simplest and most useful change theory. This theory describes systems as organizations in which "everything is related to everything else."[9] Thus, there is interdependence in a system to the extent that as one element changes another also will change.

Interdependence means that, for example, implementation of a policy in one department of a hospital will affect another department as well. Thus, if one hospital department chooses to define tardiness as "fifteen minutes late" and other departments have defined tardiness variously as "less than five minutes late," "five minutes late," and so on, all of the hospital's employees will be affected in different ways. There may be much unrest among employees in different departments in the hospital because of differences in the way they are treated.

Changes made in a system may affect elements outside of the system. When shift hours are changed from 7–3:30 P.M. to 8–4:30 P.M., family schedules must change accordingly. In both of these instances it can be seen that change does not occur in isolation.

In addition to the interdependence of elements within a system, systems theory describes a system as always in the process of seeking equilibrium. This process can be likened to the human equivalent of homeostasis. The system seeks to be stable internally and in relationship to its environment. Factors within the system itself and outside of it can affect the system's equilibrium. In industry, for example, layoffs, forced early retirement, union organizing, and strikes are examples of factors within the system that may cause instability in the system.

Factors outside of the industry that can affect its equilibrium include the state of the economy and the availability of necessary resources, both human and material. These outside factors often influence change that occurs within the system. For example, the new Occupational Safety and Health Act (OSHA) health standard on "Access to Employee Exposure and Medical Records" had an impact on industries, their employees, and occupational health nurses in relation to how access to employees' health care records was permitted and confidentiality was maintained.

In addition to understanding the process of change, the nurse must have the characteristics necessary to act as a change agent. A nurse change agent must be knowledgeable about the theory and practice of nursing. The nurse must be competent in practice. The ability to establish and maintain good interpersonal relationships is an essential characteristic of an effective change agent. Good communication skills underlie these effective human relations skills. Finally, the nurse change agent must be willing to take risks. The change, even if well planned, may not be successful, so that the nurse has to be able to take a chance and risk the consequences of failure.

Functions of the Change Agent

The nurse who is acting as a change agent has several functions. These functions, as initially described by Rogers,[10] are to:

- develop a need for the change
- diagnose the problem which exists

- design a course of action
- try out a change, and
- evaluate the change

Developing a Need for Change

A change agent often is aware of a needed change when others aren't. One of the first responsibilities of the nurse change agent is to make others equally aware of the need for the change. It may be that others are oblivious to the need for change because "It's always been done this way" and consequently, it's easier to continue doing it that way than to change. Or, it may be that others lack the knowledge to realize that the changed way of doing something is actually the better way.

The nurse must use good communication skills to make others aware of the need for change. Otherwise, trying to implement a change can be compared to "scratching where they don't itch." The nurse change agent, trying to establish the need to change a procedure, can use his or her already established networks among colleagues. The nurse might say to the other nurses on the unit "I read in the journal about a new way of catheter care involving . . . . . . What do you think about that approach?"

Here the nurse first introduces the notion that there is more than one way to do catheter care. Other nurses may not have read the same journal and so are not aware of the newer procedure.

The nurse change agent elicits the opinions of others and carefully avoids making a judgment about the worth of the procedure as it's currently being done. When others in the nurse's network also talk about the new ways of doing catheter care, the need to change the existing procedure is reinforced. Such communications will gradually expose the other nurses to the need to review the catheter care procedure, for a change may be indicated.

Diagnosing the Problem

After making others aware of the need for a change, the nurse change agent then must diagnose the problem. Problem diagnosis must be accomplished from the perspective of those with the problem. If the nurses don't want to change the catheter care procedure because it involves more work for them, changing the procedure and expecting it to be implemented won't work.

In another example, diabetic diet teaching isn't succeeding in changing a patient's eating patterns primarily because the patient's family members think he "can't possibly survive eating food like that instead of the good, home cooked kind,'' which they routinely supply for him. In this example, the nurse must try to explore the problem from the family's perspective about food if the teaching is eventually to be effective.

Problem diagnosis includes identification of the factors within and outside of the system that are related to the problem. In the preceding illustrations there are both internal and external factors that affect the problem, and ultimately the problem's solution. Once these relevant factors are identified, the nurse can sort out those that will help accomplish the change and those that will hinder the change.

Again, the nurse can benefit here from using already established networks to provide needed information. Others in his or her network can share their perspectives of the problems. They also can help identify the factors that may assist in making a change, and those that will resist change. Involvement of others in the problem diagnosis stage is more easily accomplished if the nurse has already established networks on which to rely.

An important component of diagnosing the problem from the perspective of others is the establishment of good interpersonal relationships. For the nurse change agent to be effective in problem diagnosis and resolution, he or she must have trusting relationships with those who are involved in the change process. One would assume that the nurse would have established trusting relationships with those in his or her networks. These already well-established relationships will be of value during the entire change process.

Designing a Plan for Change

When the nurse change agent has determined what the problem is, the next step is to develop a course of action to resolve the problem. Those individuals in the nurse's networks who were involved in the diagnosis of the problem also should be involved in selecting alternatives to resolve the problem. If the nurse change agent identifies the strategies for change in isolation from others who also are involved, the change will most likely be short lived.

The action plan for change must include three elements: (1) what is to be done to implement the change, (2) by whom it is to be done, and (3) by when it is to be done. The action plan identifies the strategies for change, the people who will be applying those strategies, and a target date for when the change should be accomplished.

In developing the plan for action, the nurse change agent marshals all available resources for assistance. The nurse can use resources such as professional publications, books, journals, and magazines. Human resources are available in the form of consultants and the nurse's colleagues in nursing and in other networks. Professional nursing associations also are a resource to which the nurse change agent can turn for help.

Individuals who are to be involved in the change process are helpful resources in designing the action plan. In the preceding illustrations nurses who will be implementing the new catheter care procedure should be involved in deciding how to change the current procedure to the newer one. The family members of the diabetic patient must assist the nurse in any diet teaching in order for them to become a part of the solution rather than remaining a part of the problem.

Trying Out the Change

Once the action plan has been developed, it's time to try out the change. The nurse change agent now uses effective communication skills and relies on already-established good interpersonal relationships in order to persuade others to try the change: "try it, you'll like it!" If individuals in the nurse's networks are enthusiastic about the change, they can be of tremendous assistance in encouraging others to try the change as well.

The best strategies to use in implementing a change are those that require the least adaptation on the part of the individuals involved. Strategies that are simple rather than complex are easier to try on for size. If one strategy doesn't seem to work, try another. The action plan for change should have been designed to be flexible and to include a number of strategies from which to select during the tryout period.

Getting input from others in the nurse's networks most likely will result in more strategy suggestions than the nurse could have thought of. These suggestions then can be placed in order of priority. The priorities can be based on the likelihood of their being successful strategies in implementing the change.

The nurse change agent's communication skills are used here to make the change quite apparent and visible to others in the system. Knowing that others are aware of attempts to make improvements is positive reinforcement for those trying out a change. The nurse change agent also should provide positive reinforcement for the efforts being made to change. The change will remain in effect permanently only if those who have made the change think it's a good one, and if they feel good about having made the change. Positive responses to the change by the nurse change agent and "important others" in the system can provide the necessary incentive to maintain the change.

Again, the nurse change agent here relies on members of his or her networks to help in providing this positive reinforcement. Particularly if the nurse has individuals who are in authority positions in the institution in his or her network, it should be fairly simple for the nurse to arrange for such positive feedback to be given those who are trying out the change.

Evaluating the Change

Now that the change has been tried, the final step in the process is for the nurse change agent to evaluate the change. The evaluation component does not occur only as an isolated last step in the process. Evaluation of the change process should have been occurring at every step along the way.

The nurse here attempts to determine if the change really was effective. The worth of a change is the measure of whether it accomplished what was intended. If the new catheter care procedure isn't as effective as the old one, then the change didn't really work. If nurses are doing the new procedure, but rather haphazardly because it means more work for them, then the change wasn't effective.

Timing is important in evaluating change. If the change is evaluated too soon, the effects may not be apparent, whereas a later evaluation would indicate that change did occur. It may be necessary for the nurse change agent to evaluate at intervals over a period of time to ascertain just when (and if) the change did occur.

The nurse then communicates the results of the evaluation to those involved in making the change and to the "important others" in the system. Again, the nurse uses already-established networks to help "spread the word." The networks can communicate the results of the change process throughout the institution more rapidly and effectively than the nurse can alone.

This communication reinforces the efforts of those making the change and helps to ensure that the change will be a stable one. It also reinforces the nurse's ability to effectively make changes. The tactic of broadcasting success throughout the institution by the nurse as well as the nurse's networks may result in there being less resistance when another change is to be implemented by the nurse change agent. Since the nurse has been perceived as being successful in implementing change, future change activities by that nurse also will be perceived as potentially being successful.

Resistance to Change

Even though the change is carefully planned and implemented, there most likely will be resistance. Human nature dictates that people are most comfortable with the status quo. Change is unsettling and can cause uneasiness and even pain. Individuals resist change to avoid the uncomfortable consequences of the change process.

Understanding the cause of any resistance to change is essential for the nurse change agent. Correctly identifying the cause of the resistance will help the nurse in developing strategies to overcome the resistance. The nurse can use members of his or her networks to identify causes of the resistance to change. Some of these individuals, because of their positions or experience in the institution, may be better able to identify these causes than the nurse.

Several typical causes of resistance to change are:

- the change agent himself or herself
- poor interpersonal relationships
- communication problems
- lack of understanding

The behavior of the change agent may contribute to resistance. Did he or she proceed too quickly, prematurely, ambitiously, undiplomatically? While this may be apparent to others, it often is not apparent to the change agent, who tends to blame other individuals or the system itself for the resistance.

Here, the feedback the nurse gets from members of his or her networks can be of assistance in identifying behaviors that may have adversely affected the intended change process. Feedback can help the nurse make changes in the behavior he or she exhibited that acted to hinder rather than help the change occur.

Involving others in the entire change process as much as possible is an effective strategy to overcome resistance caused by the change agent's behavior. If the change is perceived as originating only from the change agent, or if the change agent patronizes those who must change because of his or her feeling of superior knowledge, then the change will be resisted. If, however, many individuals are involved in the change, the change then belongs to the group and will be implemented as a group task, rather than as an individual task.

Does the change agent keep promises, confidences, share credit, accept responsibility for own actions? Poor interpersonal relationships will interfere with implementing a change. Others may not be willing to try something new at the encouragement of a person with whom they do not have a good relationship or whom they do not trust. Relying on already existing relationships with members of the nurse's networks should minimize the possibility that this will be a cause of resistance.

If there are poor interpersonal relationships among others who are involved in the change, there will also be difficulty in implementing a change. The nurse change agent may have to start at the level of mending existing poor interpersonal relationships before moving on to action on the change itself. If those involved with the change aren't communicating with the nurse change agent and one another, it is unlikely that the change can be implemented.

Communication always is a potential problem. The nurse has to clearly communicate to all individuals involved what the change is and the consequences of making or not making the change. All of those involved in making the change must understand the "why" of the change and the consequences if the change doesn't occur. If the nurse change agent hasn't communicated this, misunderstandings can occur that create resistance. Members of the nurse's networks can aid the nurse in communicating needed information to those involved in the change process. Again, if some of the individuals in those networks are in authority positions in the institution, communicating their support of the change to others can be of significant value.

Of course, there also can be deliberate distortions of the nurse's communications. Members of the nurse's networks can be instrumental in interpreting the nurse's communications, correcting distortions as they occur. They also can apprise the nurse when distortions are occurring, so that the nurse may take steps to remedy the situation. This form of resistance has to be dealt with immediately when it occurs if the change is to succeed.

Lack of understanding about the change process, either on the part of the nurse change agent or others, can cause resistance. The nurse who fails to adequately plan to accommodate elements outside, as well as inside, the system demonstrates a lack of understanding of the interdependence of elements which can cause change to fail. For example, the nurse who considers only the diabetic patient's nutritional needs and "food likes and dislikes" but fails to consider the "outside" element of his family's influence will not be likely to change his current eating patterns.

There can be lack of understanding on the part of the individuals involved in the change. They may not really understand how the change will improve their current situation and so may prefer the status quo.

Resistance to change may be either active or passive. The active forms of resistance are easier to recognize, such as the deliberate distortion of the nurse change agent's communication. This active resistance must be dealt with immediately. Confrontation is usually the technique of choice.

The nurse must exercise caution not to become angry during the confrontation. The purpose of the confrontation should be to elicit reasons for the person's actions so that steps may be taken to minimize the influence of this disruption. It may well be that the individual does not understand the need for the change, and his or her perception of the change is threatening. The nurse should deal with the causes of the active resistance quietly but firmly.

Passive forms of resistance are harder to identify and to deal with. Individuals who feel they lack the power to "make a difference" often resort to passive resistance to accomplish their aims. Such resistance may be exhibited in procrastination or delay in following orders. Again, involving as many individuals as possible in the entire change process will help eliminate the feeling of powerlessness and will increase the feeling that the change belongs to them, thus decreasing resistance.

Change that is initiated from inside the system generally causes less resistance than change from outside the system. Outsiders are perceived as knowing less about the system than those who work within it.

In contrast, recommendations for change from outside the system often get more action from those in authority than changes recommended by individuals inside the system. This is perhaps accounted for because outsiders are supposed to have a "more objective" viewpoint than those inside the system. Most outside recommendations for change come from those who are perceived to have a legitimate right to make such recommendations, such as accreditation visitors, consultants, and so on.

Overcoming Resistance

The nurse change agent must be skilled in overcoming resistance to change. Careful, methodical planning for change will tend to reduce the amount of resistance, but may not entirely eliminate it. As resistance is encountered it must be analyzed for its cause and for probable strategies that would be effective to overcome it.

The nurse change agent has to be flexible when resistance is encountered. Adhering rigidly to the notion that the change must happen in a specific way will increase resistance and defeat the nurse change agent's ultimate purpose. The entire process must be viewed as open to changes by everyone involved. The nurse has to be able to accommodate suggested modifications if the need arises.

The ability to understand the fears and concerns of those who are in the process of changing will help the nurse change agent minimize resistance. If those involved in the resistance were part of the planning for change process, they can be involved in planning to overcome the resistance as well.

POWER

Power is defined by the *Random House College Dictionary* as the "ability to do or act; capability of doing or accomplishing something." That definition certainly is innocuous, yet, traditionally, power has not been an acceptable topic for discussion, at least not in nursing circles. Describing someone, particularly a woman, as "power hungry" was a cruel epithet. But here is another side of the coin: not using power when you have it and when you need to also is unnecessary cruelty—and you are the victim. Of itself, power is neutral. What is negative or positive is the way power is used by individuals, not the power itself. Women, and nurses as well, need to understand the uses—and the abuses—of power.

Understanding power begins with understanding the relationship between power and authority. Authority generally refers to the legitimate right of an individual to issue orders or directives and expect them to be obeyed. Power is the force or influence one commands. Illegitimate power can be described as the issuance of orders or directives without the authority to do so.

One can view this relationship in the context of an illustration in which a hospital administrator develops a new policy on employee absenteeism. Because he has the authority to make such a policy based on his status in the organization and the legitimate rights of his position, he expects that all employees will follow the policy to the letter. When employees are absent, the administrator can use his power to discipline them for not following the policy. The discipline can range from verbal warnings to dismissal if the severity of the infractions warrant.

This is an example of legitimate power. However, not all power is legitimate. In a group meeting, for example, where the topic of employee absenteeism is the subject under discussion, the hospital administrator may indicate that he expects the policy to be strictly enforced. The head of one department disagrees, citing as an example an employee in his department who is frequently absent but for whom there are "extenuating circumstances." During the discussion, others side with this department head, with the end result being that the group decides the policy will be strictly enforced only when they wish it to be. The department head here wielded power that was not legitimate but that had more influence over the members of the group than the legitimate power of the hospital administrator.

Power is essential for healthy functioning of an individual. It is the feeling of powerlessness, whether real or not, that leads to frustration and to the now common "burn-out" of nurses. There are ways that can help you build your power base. Among these are to:

- identify your professional and personal strengths
- identify your weaknesses and deficiencies
- use your strengths in ways that will be successful and that will minimize your weaknesses and deficiencies
- build support systems (networks) for yourself
- solicit feedback from your support systems (networks) about any successes or any failures in your attempts to use your power

It also is important to recognize when you have power. The power you have can be your legitimate right, based on your position in an institution or organization. In that case, the power is known as "formal" power. Or, the power you have can be based on individual factors, because of your influence with others. In that case, the power is described as "informal" power.

When you exert your influence over others—when you get someone to do what you want—you are exercising your power. Because power easily can be exercised for the wrong purposes, it is equally as important to recognize the abuse of power. In an article in *Nursing Management,* noted attorney Aaron Levenstein describes the several forms of power originally classified by the psychologist Rollo May.[11] These types of power are:

- exploitative
- manipulative
- competitive
- nutrient
- integrative

Power that exploits others is abusive. In this circumstance the individual is not treated as a person. Those who use power in this manner overlook the rights of the individual.

The exercise of power that attempts to have one individual accommodate the wishes of another, when those wishes may not be in his or her best interests, is manipulative. Often, such power is exercised through deception.

Competitive power is that which is exercised in instances where many individuals want to reach the same goal, although only one or a few are able to attain that goal. This power is evidenced when resources must be shared by many. For example, when there are limited funds for new equipment in an institution and all departments must bid for their share of the equipment, there generally is competition. In this instance, those who wield the most power, whether formal or informal, are likely to end up with the greater share of equipment funds.

This form of power can be abusive to others or not, depending, of course, on the individuals who exercise the power. The exercise of competitive power can be constructive or destructive.

Power that takes into consideration the other individual's best interests is called nutrient power. Here one individual uses his or her influence to assist another. This is the power illustrated by making referrals in the process of networking. An individual who refers someone in his or her network to another is using nutrient power.

Integrative power also is used in networking. This form of power, according to Levenstein, initially was described by May as "power with the other person."[12] In using integrative power, an individual exercises influence to assist another individual in taking advantage of opportunities to grow both personally and professionally. An individual who is serving as a mentor uses integrative power as he or she is instrumental in aiding the person being mentored to progress.

In order to network effectively, and to grow professionally, nurses first must know how to increase their power. Equally important is for nurses to recognize that they have power. Finally, nurses must know what type of power they have and how to use their power effectively.

SUMMARY

There are many strategies to assist the nurse to grow professionally. Initially, of course, the nurse must set his or her professional goals. In order to know if professional growth has occurred, the nurse must begin by deciding where he or she expects to go, so that it will be easy to assess progress. Once professional goals are set, strategies such as knowing how to be assertive and how to use power are essential. Being skilled in implementing change in situations where the status quo does not facilitate the nurse's attainment of his or her professional goals is another strategy that must be in the nurse's behavioral repertoire.

An essential element of all of these strategies for professional growth of the nurse is networking. Whether learning to be assertive, and getting feedback on improvements in assertive behavior, or involving others in implementing a needed change, or influencing others through the exercise of power for the purpose of getting what nurses want, networking can be an effective tool for nurses to use.

Nurses can use their networking skills within and outside the nursing profession. Nurses can network with one another and with those in other health care professions in order to achieve their own personal goals as well as their professional goals.

Nurses can network to change positions, to take advantage of professional opportunities, to make an impact on the political arena, or to improve their economic and general welfare. Nurses can network not only to meet their professional goals as individuals, but they also can influence the future directions of the nursing profession through their networking.

The rich heritage of the profession can be passed along through nurses mentoring one another. Young men and women can be socialized into the profession through networking. Nurses working together to influence the direction nursing takes in the future is a thrilling prospect. Nurses using their networking skills to help themselves, other nurses, and the profession as a whole can help make that exciting vision a reality.

NOTES

1. Sidney B. Simon, Leland W. Howe, and Howard Kirschenbaum, *Values Clarification* (New York: Hart,1972), p. 12.

2. Janet Stone and Jane Bachner, *Speaking Up* (New York: McGraw-Hill, 1977), p. xiii.

3. Ibid., pp. 10–31.

4. Ibid., pp. 32–55.

5. Elizabeth Janeway, *Man's World, Woman's Place: A Study in Social Mythology* (New York: Dell, 1971), p. 7.

6. Melodie Chenevert, *Special Techniques in Assertiveness Training* (St. Louis: C.V. Mosby, 1978), p. 39.

7. Belinda E. Puetz, "Who Cares for the Care-Givers?", *Occupational Health Nursing,* October, 1981, pp. 34–37

8. Ingeborg G. Mauksch and Michael H. Miller, *Implementing Change in Nursing* (St. Louis: C.V. Mosby, 1981), p. 9.

9. L.F. Thompson, M.H. Miller, and H.F. Bigler, *Sociology: Nurses and Their Patients in Modern Society* (St. Louis: C.V. Mosby, 1975), p. 7.

10. E.M. Rogers, "Change Agents, Clients and Change," in *Creating Social Change,* ed. G. Zaltman, P. Kotter, and I. Kaufman (New York: Holt, Rinehart & Winston, 1972), pp. 196–197.

11. Aaron Levenstein, "The Uses of Power," *Nursing Management* 12, no. 10 (October 1981): 24–25.

12. Ibid., p. 25.

Index

About the Author

BELINDA E. PUETZ, R.N., Ph.D., is Administrator, Education and Practice Programs, Indiana State Nurses' Association, Indianapolis, Indiana, and Assistant Professor, School of Nursing, Indiana University. Dr. Puetz also is the founder of the consulting firm Continuing Education Unlimited. Currently, Dr. Puetz is a member of the executive committee of the American Nurses' Association Council on Continuing Education.